THE **FARMHOUSE CULTURE GUIDE** TO

FERMENTING

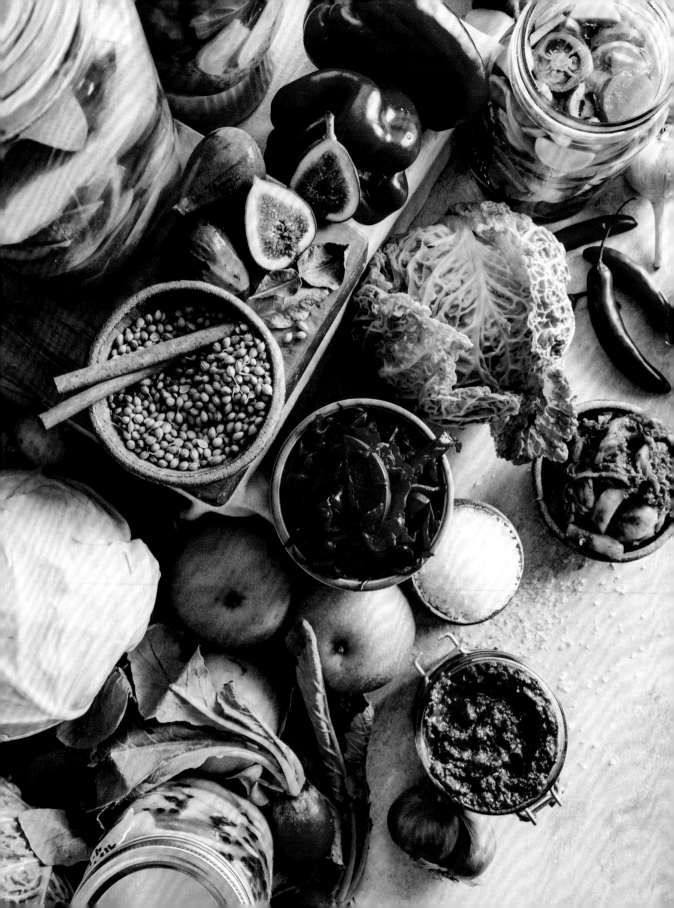

KATHRYN LUKAS & SHANE PETERSON

THE **FARMHOUSE CULTURE GUIDE** TO
FERMENTING

Crafting Live-Cultured Foods and Drinks with
100 Recipes from Kimchi to Kombucha

PHOTOGRAPHS BY ERIC WOLFINGER

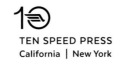

TEN SPEED PRESS
California | New York

To all of our friends, family, and employees
who helped breathe life into Farmhouse Culture.

Contents

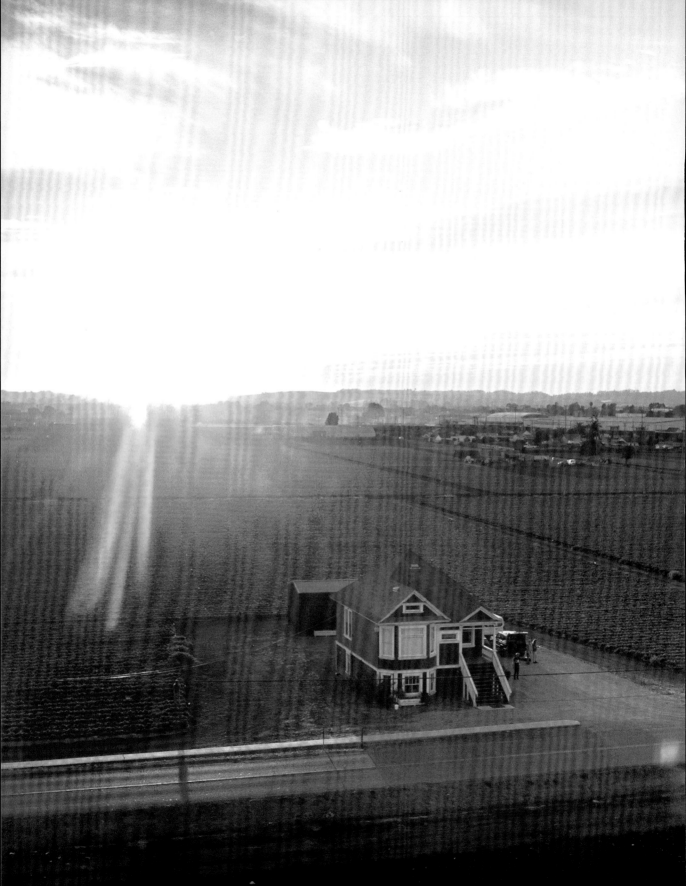

THE
Farmhouse Culture Story

When I reflect back on all the factors leading up to 2008, it seems as though my entire life's journey had been in preparation for Farmhouse Culture, and it all started with my grandparents' farmhouse. Grandpa John, who owned the Guadalupe Mines in Los Gatos, California, and a small cattle ranch and walnut orchard in Gridley, California, was a larger-than-life Irishman who loved to eat (and drink), and my grandmother, Lillian, was happy to oblige him. My sister, mother, and I lived with my grandparents in Los Gatos for most of my childhood, but summers were spent at the ranch in Gridley. It was there in our old white farmhouse that I came to understand the connection between Grandpa John's gardens and animals, and what landed on our plates. Both my grandparents cooked, but it was Grandpa who was the family preservationist. He canned every-thing, from dilly beans and tomatoes to grape jelly, and the entire family was required to pitch in. With every jar opened throughout the year, the memory of those raucous family gatherings, full of laughter, intense aromas, and sticky fingers, fortified our meals with deep satisfaction.

As I was tossing around names for my budding little sauerkraut com-pany, I kept thinking back to my family's farmhouse and my memories of how ingredients were lovingly transformed into healthful and delicious foods. Although my first products were sauerkrauts (because it was a famil-iar food for most Americans), I knew from the beginning that I wanted to eventually introduce many more traditional live-culture foods and bever-ages, and the name "Farmhouse Culture" provided the girth needed to expand. Yes, I thought, this would be a fine name for my new company, while honoring the care, lessons, and love my grandparents so generously shared with me. And it might even make up for breaking Grandpa John's heart when I became a vegetarian.

It was my quirky Norwegian grandmother, Roxanne, who was convinced that my fiery teenage energy could be tamed with a vegetarian, macro-biotic diet. A free-spirited nonconformist, she was deeply distrustful of the corporate food system and in the 1960s had found her way to brown rice, whole-wheat bread, and tofu. She swore the new diet helped with her arthritis and might even save the world. It was in her wise care, and with her "hippie" foods, that I not only calmed down, but also fell in love with cooking. Grandma Roxanne taught me that knowing how to cook healthy foods was the ultimate form of rebellion, and that if one was going attempt to make the world a better place, a healthy body and a strong mind were absolute necessities. She lit the fire that still burns strong in my belly today.

Falling in love with a German and moving to Stuttgart, Germany, in my late twenties was another defining moment on the road to sauerkraut. At our restaurant, Das Augustenstüble, I learned to cook the regional Schwäbisch cuisine and to love canned sauerkraut—if it was properly prepared. Rinsed well; braised with apples, onions, and duck fat; and doused with wine, it was a huge improvement over the straight-out-of-the-can stuff Grandpa John served with hot dogs. But it wasn't until a trip to a farm outside Stuttgart to refill our schnapps bucket for the restaurant that I discovered an even better version. Our visits had become an anticipated and delicious monthly ritual. The farmer, Herr Lutz, was a jolly and boisterous fellow and always eager to share the foods and drinks he and his wife worked so hard to grow and prepare. Normally there were things like apricots and plums and new flavors of schnapps, so I wasn't totally prepared when Herr Lutz handed me a forkful of sauerkraut from a large wooden barrel. Still assuming that straight sauerkraut tasted like the canned kraut I was familiar with, I was hesitant, but of course I couldn't refuse. I inhaled deeply and prepared for the onslaught of that intense salty sourness I had come to expect. But instead, I experienced a mild, pleasing tanginess and a slight herbaceousness, followed by just a hint of vegetal sweetness. The briny finish brought all the flavors together into a gorgeous and harmonious taste. This was something entirely different than canned sauerkraut, and I was immediately smitten. Herr Lutz provided me with a little history and a quick kraut how-to lesson, but it wasn't until many years later in Santa Cruz that I actually made my first batch of sauerkraut.

I returned home to California in 1998, single and heartbroken. Over the next few years I worked in hospitality management, but eventually became restless. After so many years working with mostly Northern European haute cuisine, I had also become bored—I was itching to travel, to learn about new foods, and to cook again. Fascinated with vegan, raw, and traditional folk preparation techniques, I was also feeling nostalgic for the healthier foods from my grandmother's kitchen, and in 2004, the Natural Chef Training Program at Bauman College in Santa Cruz seemed like a great place to start my journey back to cooking.

While there, I learned for the first time about digestive health. Donna Gate's book *The Body Ecology Diet* was required reading. One of the earliest nutritionists to use the terms *leaky gut* and *inner ecosystem*, her protocol to rid the digestive system of gut-disrupting candida yeast included ½ cup of raw cultured vegetables per day. In Germany, it was generally assumed that sauerkraut was healthy, and I noticed that the Germans drank the brine when they were hungover, but I'd never thought of it as a "health food." In my world, sauerkraut had simply been an excellent culinary ingredient and condiment. I was intrigued, and could hardly contain my enthusiasm the day we made our first batch. We massaged salt into chopped cabbage, tucked it into a small fermenting crock, and waited. Over the next few days, the crock literally came alive with sounds and smells. We could it hear it gurgling and burping as we worked on other projects in the kitchen, and the sulfurous aroma intensified by the day. By the time we peeked inside, a couple of weeks later, the bubbling had subsided and a sweet, earthy aroma greeted us. Our instructor plunged her gloved hand into the crock and pulled out a mass of glossy cabbage shreds for us to sample. In a split second I was blasted back to Herr Lutz's cellar, tasting that first revelatory bite of fresh kraut, and I was hooked.

At the time, Sandor Ellix Katz's *Wild Fermentation* was the go-to book for novice fermenters, but within the first few pages, I realized that it was much more than a fermentation manual: it was also a treatise on how to reclaim our food system and our health, and it spoke to something deep inside my soul. Right alongside my desire to learn a new food craft was a deepening frustration with the American food system. After experiencing the joy of regionally specific foods made by multigenerational food artisans in Europe, American cuisine felt shallow to me. Restaurant food, at the time mostly served up by chains, tasted the same whether you were in Boston or San Francisco, and much of the food found at grocery stores was overprocessed and filled with unpronounceable ingredients. Obesity was climbing at an alarming rate, and nutritionists were calling for bland low-fat diets to counter the trend. None of this felt right to me. I was drawn to the rich cultural history of traditional foods, and if rebelling against these strange new American food norms was a road map to a better world, then I was in. I know Grandma Roxanne would have approved.

Following pages: Farmhouse Culture's cabbage suppliers, Lakeside Organic Gardens in Watsonville, California

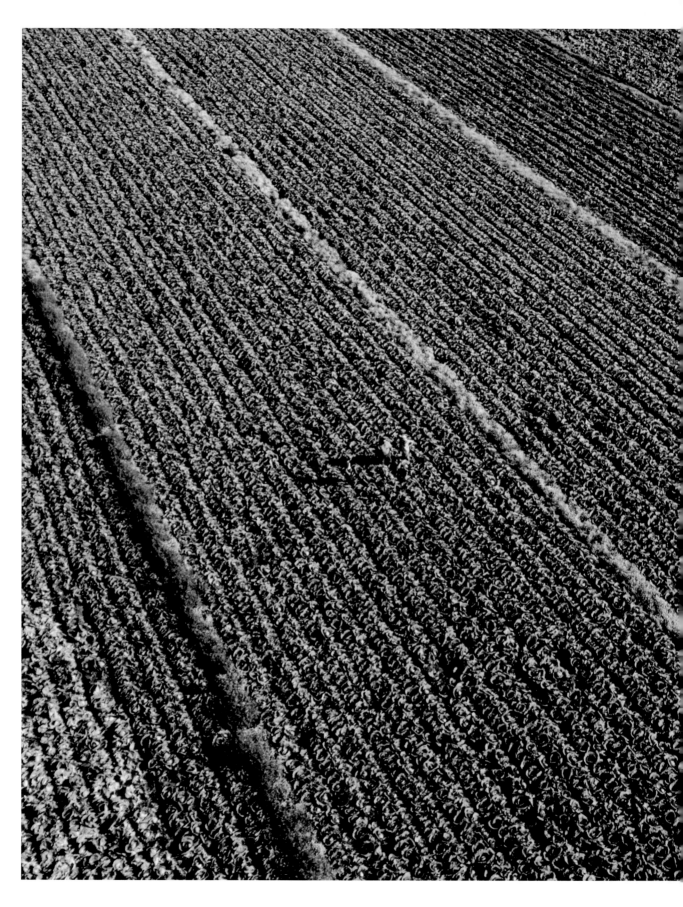

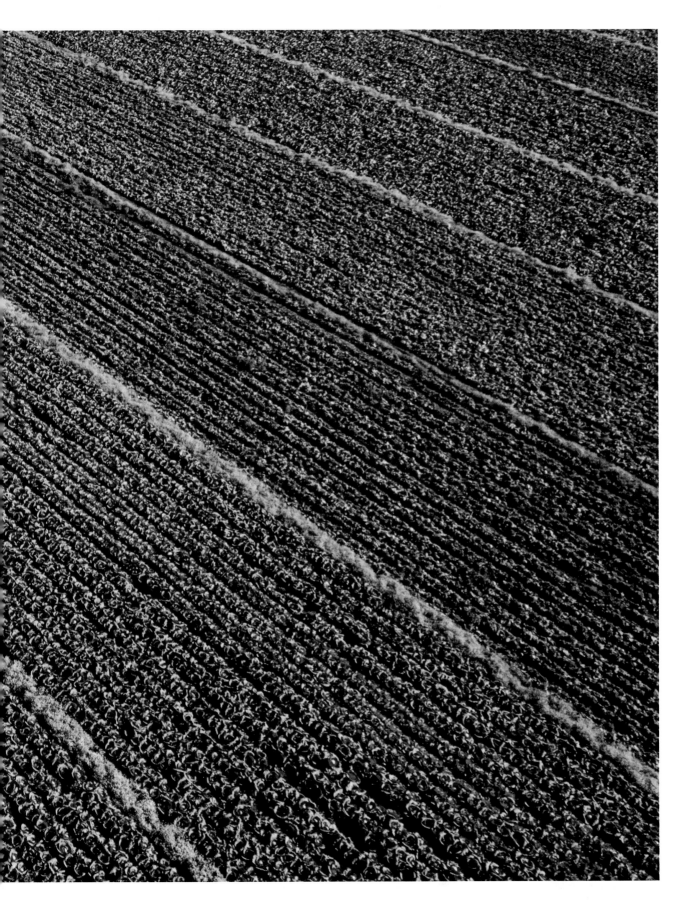

I dug into Katz's book with a religious fervor and discovered a hidden world of microbes that miraculously transformed ordinary ingredients, like cabbage, into superfoods. Sauerkraut was just the beginning. Crocks of pungent kimchi and chunky misos took over the closet in my spare room, and my counters were crowded with half-gallon jars of kombucha, kvass, and water kefir. My home felt alive with the sound of bubbling and the unfamiliar aromas, and I felt like a painter who had suddenly discovered a whole new spectrum of colors. As each new flavor emerged, I began imagining how it would taste paired with various ingredients and where it would best fit into a meal. Once I was comfortable with a basic formula, I would start tinkering with new ingredients, fermentation times, and temperatures just to see what was possible. There were plenty of slimy, skunky disasters, but there were also triumphs, and as my repertoire of recipes grew, I realized that I had found something more than a new craft: I had found my calling.

In a small cabin that overlooked a pond just outside Yosemite in Groveland, California, Farmhouse Culture was born. An opportunity to escape the bustle of the Bay Area for a few months had come up and the break afforded me the time and space I needed to dream and think my new business idea into life. The community was enthusiastically supportive, and soon I had hatched a plan with my new friends, farmers Christine and Eric Taylor, to turn their cabbage into sauerkraut for their CSA box. Our landlords, Ellie and Patricia (who were also our neighbors), offered their kitchen and cool basement for those very first batches of sauerkraut.

It was also during this time that I became interested in the Slow Food movement and joined a local chapter. My heart skipped a beat at one of the meetings when I saw a flyer for an upcoming event in San Francisco called Slow Food Nation. They were looking for regional growers and food artisans to showcase their goods at a farmers' market that would be set up in the city center for the event. Having recently learned that Slow Food had a catalog of traditional foods at risk of going extinct, called the Ark of Taste, and that fresh, unpasteurized sauerkraut was on the list, I knew immediately that this was the right event to introduce my fresh krauts to the Bay Area. A few days later, not wanting to take any chances with the July heat, I drove to San Francisco and hand-delivered my Classic Caraway, Apple a Day, and Holy Smokes sauerkrauts to the Slow Food Nation office. A couple of weeks later, when a letter arrived announcing that my Holy Smokes sauerkraut had been accepted, I danced and yippee'd and hollered with joy.

And then I got to work; I had exactly five weeks to get 1,500 pounds of cabbage and smoked jalapeños into barrels and fermenting, and I wasn't entirely sure I could pull it off.

Three days before the event, a blistering heat wave descended on Groveland. As the thermostat outside climbed to 107°F, I could feel the last bit of cool air being sucked out of my neighbors' basement. In desperation, we resorted to filling large trash bags with ice and taping them to the barrels, but the ice melted faster than we could replenish it. The internal temperature of the sauerkraut peaked at a still-safe 75°F, but that was twenty degrees more than I wanted. In tears, I thought seriously about canceling. How could I debut sauerkraut that was less than perfect to a discerning Slow Food crowd? My friends reassured me that the kraut still tasted quite good and urged me to reconsider. Still feeling very unsure, I took a deep breath and decided to go for it.

The next morning, I packed the Holy Smokes sauerkraut I had made for the event into my van, along with the three barrels I had made for the Taylors' CSA. Refrigeration was their only chance of surviving at this point, and I figured I could bring back whatever we didn't use. My friends had been right. Not only was the Holy Smokes acceptable, it was met with rave reviews. Long lines, six people deep, formed on Friday, and remained in place until we ran out on Sunday afternoon. By the time the event was over, we had handed out over eight thousand samples and sold everything I had made for the season. That damned heat wave had turned out to be a blessing.

Exhilarated and bolstered by the enthusiastic reception at Slow Food Nation, I decided it was time to move home to Santa Cruz and start a fresh fermented sauerkraut business in earnest. I fleshed out my business plan, worked on a package design, and found several local farmers who could provide the gorgeous vegetables that would soon fill my barrels. By February 2009, I had moved into a beautiful production facility, and not long after, I recruited my son and a couple of willing friends and together we made our first barrel of sauerkraut. By May, we were selling our fresh sauerkrauts at the Santa Cruz Community Farmers' Market and then soon after at local California grocers such as New Leaf and Staff of Life. Whole Foods approached us before we could catch our breath, and suddenly we were selling our krauts nationwide.

Farmhouse Culture was very much a family affair in the beginning. My sister Julianne, who had helped out at Slow Food Nation, worked at our farmers' market booths and special events, and did a bit of bookkeeping and HR. My brother-in-law, Jason, gave up a job of ten years to help make sauerkraut and manage what would eventually grow to fourteen weekly farmers' market booths. Jason's father, John Lindsay, had been the editor at the *Santa Cruz Sentinel* for more than twenty years and knew everyone in town. He'd show up at our Santa Cruz farmers' markets with his cowboy hat and handlebar mustache, and entice customers into our booth for a taste. John was also our plumber, carpenter, electrician, and psychologist, and soon he was known simply as "the Bürgermeister," the German word for "mayor." With their love and energy, the business grew faster than any of us could have imagined.

When I started the business, my son, Shane, helped when he could, but was still pretty convinced that a career as a professional golfer was his path. He bartended by night, played tournaments by day, and worked for us in production and at special events and farmers' markets part-time. As much as I wanted him to come to work for Farmhouse Culture full-time, I understood and supported his golfing dream. I secretly hoped that one day he would change his mind, and that perhaps the love of gardening and good food his Grandpa Jack and I had instilled in him early on might somehow bring him into the fold.

In 2011, my wish started to come true. After attending a life-changing indigenous skills retreat in Mount Shasta, Shane decided he wanted to live closer to the land and migrated from his place in town to our property in the Soquel hills. He planted a big garden and started wandering and foraging in the redwood forests that bordered our land.

And then disaster struck. On my birthday in March 2012, Shane was in a serious car accident that required an airlift to a head trauma unit in San Jose. For three of the longest hours of my life, I had no idea if he would survive, and to this day, I can't think about that time without a lump in my throat. Shane turned out to be a very, very lucky man. His head injuries were not severe, and he was able to return home fairly quickly.

After a month of recuperating, Shane emerged from his cocoon a changed man with a new passion for homesteading. He quit his job bartending, went to work for Mountain Feed & Farm Supply, and decided that golf would become a hobby. I'd never seen him so possessed. By early summer, our gardens were bursting with vegetables, we had huge compost piles (another form of fermentation) and worm bins, and ten chickens had moved to the property, along with three beehives. Shane was now milking our neighbor's goats on a regular basis and making his own cheese and yogurt. His foraging resulted in blackberry jams, elderberry syrups, and herbal hand salves. When his garden exploded with Kirby cucumbers that he had planted in order to make pickles, his interest in fermentation went from being "mom's thing" to an important part of his now thriving homestead. The half-sour pickles he made that season were the best any of us had ever tasted. I'm not sure if it was his treasured compost pile or those amazing pickles, but by the end of that summer, he had fallen hard for fermentation.

Shane brought his newfound fervor to Farmhouse Culture, and soon he was wearing multiple hats like the rest of us. Farmers' markets, special events, sales, trade shows, production—he did it all, but it was becoming clear that his talent and true love was in the science of fermentation and creating new products. When we finally had a real innovation department, Shane became our head fermentologist. His knowledge of fermentation and his passion for sharing that knowledge deepened even further when the opportunity came up to write a book about fermentation for a Danish publisher with his good friend Søren Ejlersen, which became a bestseller in Denmark.

Between my obsession with flavor and Shane's fascination and knowledge of all things fermented, we make a pretty good team. It doesn't hurt that we've been cooking together since Shane was old enough to push a chair up to the kitchen counter, so when the time came to write this book, we knew we had to write it together. Our goal for the book is simple: share our love of fermentation and our hard-won knowledge so that you can create the most delicious and healthful ferments possible.

Happy Fermenting,

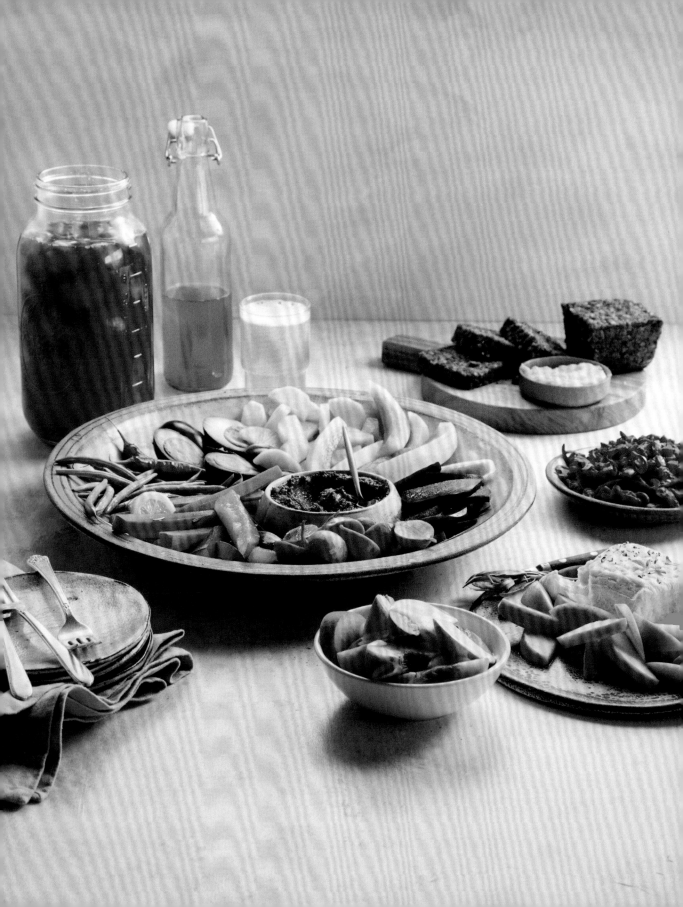

THE
Fermentation Story

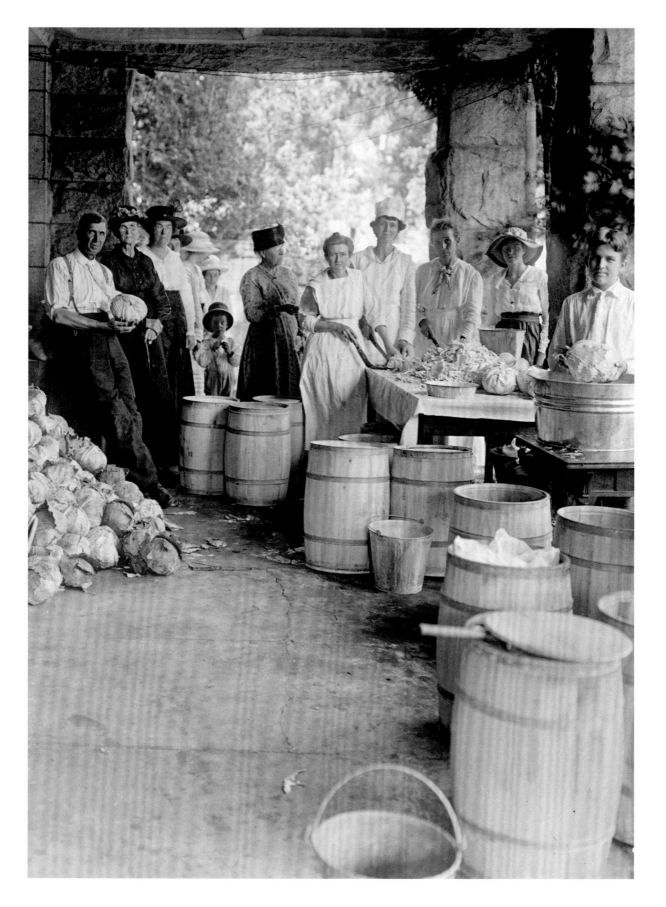

In this chapter, we'll take you on a whirlwind tour through the history of fermentation, the most ancient of preservation techniques, and then do our best to help you understand how these foods came to be cherished and why they are so critically beneficial to human health. We'll also provide a broad overview of the science of fermentation before taking a deeper dive into the various types of ferments explored later in this book. Don't worry if science isn't your thing or if all the information doesn't sink in at once. You'll have plenty of opportunity to learn as you go. We're confident that our detailed recipes will guide you to success regardless of your scientific aptitude, and we're pretty sure the microbes will be conspiring behind the scenes to aid you as well.

The Wild History of Fermentation

It's hard for historians to pinpoint exactly when humans began an active partnership with microbial fermentation because, much like fire, fermentation was a discovery rather than an invention. We don't know, for instance, how long it took humans to figure out that they could make mead, the mind-altering drink made from honeycombs that had come in contact with water, widely considered one of the first fermented beverages. But it's safe to say that our ability to observe, understand, and eventually manipulate the fermentation of plants and animals is inextricably linked to our success as a species, and the development of human culture. And speaking of "culture," isn't it fascinating that we use this word to describe both the collection of things people make when they come together, like literature, music, painting, and philosophy, as well as the community of microbes used to ferment food and drink?

Making sauerkraut
in North Carolina, 1917.

The word *culture* comes from the Latin *cultura*, and from *colere*, which means "to tend, guard, till, cultivate." Although the earliest records indicate that human-controlled fermentation predates agriculture, the cultivation of land necessitated the acceleration of the craft so surplus crops could be preserved. A good fermented beverage may have also been a motivating factor; some anthropologists even speculate that agriculture was first conceived so humans could procure a steadier supply of alcohol. There certainly does seem to be a connection between imbibing and great works of art. In fact, Horace said, "No poems can please long or live that are written by water-drinkers."

Many of the formulas in this book rely on salt to kick-start a fermentation process that favors a community of bacteria called lactobacilli, and is commonly referred to as lacto-fermentation. Historians speculate that one of the earliest salt ferments of the ancient world may have originated in Rome, where fish scraps were fermented into a thick, dark sauce called *garum*. It appears that at about the same time, a similar sauce called *jiang* was popular in Southeast Asia. The Chinese added soybeans to the ferment and later eliminated the fish, calling their version *jiangyou*, better known today as soy sauce.[1] Coastal Mediterranean foragers in Asia during the primitive pottery age (8000 to 3000 BCE) stored vegetables in seawater in large pots, which produced the earliest versions of kimchi, the Korean-style cabbage ferment.[2] The domestication of cattle in the Middle East around the same time likely led to dairy ferments such as cheese and yogurt. Next came cucumbers, which are thought to have been first fermented around 2000 BCE in the Middle East, and are also mentioned several times in the Christian Bible.[3] The European-style sauerkraut most of us are familiar with was transported by the Mongols in their thirteenth-century invasions of Central Europe.

We may have first employed fermentation to alter our state of consciousness and preserve food, but it couldn't have taken long to comprehend that the process also created incredibly compelling flavors. I am awed by those early fermenters, whose ingenuity and persistence helped to create so many of the foods and drinks we cherish. Sourdough bread, cheese, certain cured meats, chocolate, coffee, vanilla, soy sauce, miso, olives, sauerkraut, pickles, beer, wine, spirits—this is just a sampling of the thousands of fermented products available worldwide. In fact, fermentation is still employed to produce as much as a third of the world's foods.

1 Mark Kurlansky, *Salt: A World History* (London: Walker Books, 2002), 20.

2 Fred Breidt, Roger F. McFeeters, Ilenys Perez-Diaz, and Cherl-Ho Lee, "Fermented Vegetables," in M. P. Doyle and R. L. Buchanan, eds., *Food Microbiology: Fundamentals and Frontiers*, 4th ed. (Washington, DC: ASM Press, 2013), 841–55, https://fbns.ncsu.edu/USDAARS/Acrobatpubs/P376-400/p380.pdf.

3 Breidt et al., "Fermented Vegetables."

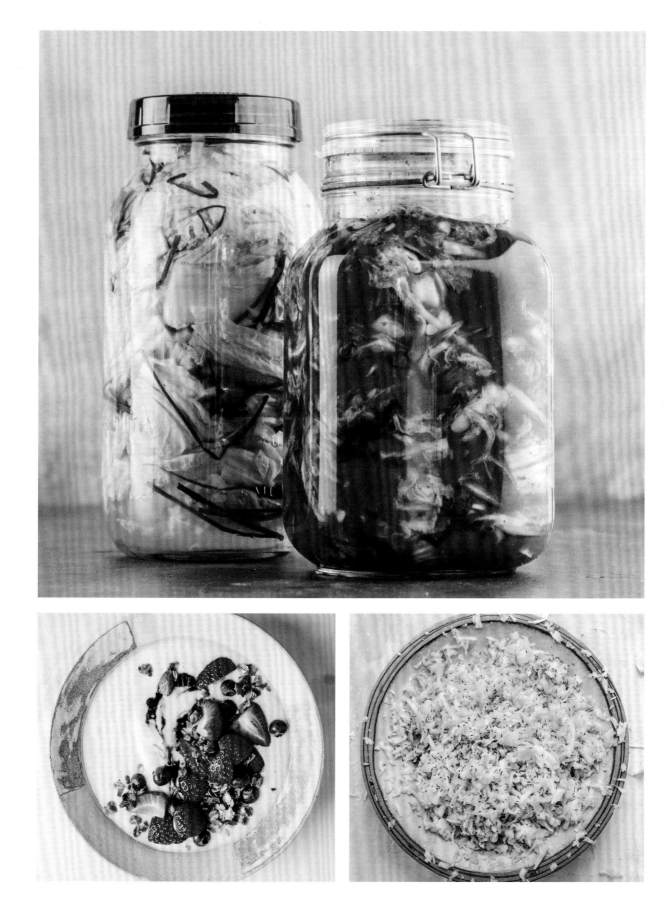

There is a distinction, though, between a fermented food and a ferment that retains live cultures. While all live-cultured foods are fermented, not all fermented foods that end up on your plate are alive. For example, fermentation is employed in the processing of many foods such as chocolate, bread, and coffee to enhance flavor, give rise, or neutralize harmful phytonutrients, but they do not retain live cultures. With very few exceptions, the recipes in this book are "alive" with the ancient microbes that we humans have coevolved with over millennia.

Unfortunately, the war on bacteria over the last century has resulted in a radical shift in our perception of live-culture foods, and many of these beloved foods and beverages have either disappeared or been replaced with sterile versions. Although Louis Pasteur's research on germ theory saved countless lives, it also led to the belief that all microbes are "germs" and should be feared and eradicated. As a result, many of us grew up completely unaware of live-culture foods. Canned sauerkraut was simply, well, sauerkraut. Perhaps it would have been different if we all had grown up in the Midwest, where many families still make homemade sauerkraut, or in New York City, where pickle and sauerkraut shops were once abundant.

At the turn of the twentieth century, there were more than eighty such shops and carts on New York's Lower East Side, but when I (Kathryn) visited the neighborhood in 2008, only one shop remained: Guss' Pickles. Rather than the "pickle emporium" full of tourists that I had imagined, the tiny basement shop was barely noticeable from the street. I was met with a gruff "hey" by a guy in a royal blue smock giving a sample to the shop's lone customer, who was clearly a local. When it was my turn, I sampled everything, from the full- and half-sour pickles to a strange, sweet sauerkraut from a big blue barrel. Curious about the sweet kraut, I asked the sample guy how it was sweetened. "I put my finger in it!" he bellowed before breaking into a deep belly laugh. A year later, Guss' closed their Lower East Side shop and moved to Brooklyn. I still smile when I think of my visit, and am glad I was able to experience the last of the great Lower East Side pickle and kraut shops. Sadly, during the twentieth century, nearly all these types of shops were replaced by large-scale production where pasteurization is the norm. But a health renaissance that would breathe life back into sauerkraut and pickles was around the corner.

In the 1960s, a hippie exodus to rural communities in the US and Canada was under way. Educated and determined, these hardy souls learned self-sufficiency from scratch. They took Rachel Carson's 1962 environmental treatise *Silent Spring* seriously, and not long after, with the help of J. I. Rodale, birthed the organic farming movement. (Perhaps not coincidentally, Rodale was from New York's Lower East Side.) These back-to-the-land communities experimented with communal living, became vegetarians, and created food cooperatives (many of which still exist). Their interest in wholesome, unprocessed foods, like brown rice, tofu, naturally leavened breads, and fresh sauerkraut, represented much more than nourishment. It was a response to the tumultuous times, the Vietnam War, and the food corporations whose dead, overprocessed foods had come to symbolize everything that was wrong with our culture.

Perhaps it's no surprise, then, that the godfather of modern fermentation, Sandor Ellix Katz, found his inspiration in a back-to-the-land community in rural Tennessee. Originally from Manhattan's Upper West Side, Katz grew up loving the garlicky sour pickles from Zabar's but didn't "find" fermentation until a bumper crop of cabbage and radishes found him. I (Kathryn) first met Katz at our booth at Slow Food Nation in San Francisco on Labor Day weekend in 2008, and like a giddy schoolgirl, I could hardly contain my excitement. When he declared my Smoked Jalapeño kraut "delicious," I thought I had died and gone to heaven. His first book, *Wild Fermentation*, demystified fermentation for an entire generation of eager fermenters, but it went further than instruction and a handful of recipes. Katz helped us make the connection between the microbes in the soil, the crock, and our guts, and outlined how making a quart of sauerkraut could help heal this ancient relationship and, ultimately, heal ourselves and the planet. In the book's foreword, nutritionist Sally Fallon Morrell captured the spirit of the people drawn to the movement:

> *Wild Fermentation* represents not only an effort to bring back from oblivion these treasured processes but also a road map to a better world, a world of healthy people and equitable economies, a world that especially values those iconoclastic, free thinking individuals—so often labeled misfits—uniquely qualified to perform the alchemy of fermented foods.

We "fermentos" were part of something bigger than ourselves; we were part of a movement that was fueling a cultural revival, both microbial and human, and we all believed the world would be a better place for it. It turns out, we might have been right.

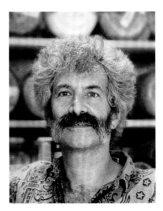

THE PHILOSOPHER KRAUT KING, SANDOR ELLIX KATZ

Why do you think live-culture foods have become so popular in recent years?

I think we're seeing an explosion of interest specifically in raw, unpasteurized, live-cultured foods because the term *microbiome* has become a household word and has changed the popular perception of bacteria. People see the promise of probiotic bacteria and the importance of restoring the biodiversity of the gut to improve digestion, immune function, mental health, and more.

What do you think is next for live-culture ferments?

There is a lot of innovation happening right now, a lot of sharing of new ideas and information, and I find this really exciting. Hopefully, interest will continue to grow, and the kinds of commercial products will continue to diversify so people don't think fermentation means kombucha, or that one singular food doesn't become representative of the whole phenomenon. I believe that the power of probiotics is all about diversity and eating as many different types of foods as possible.

The New Frontier

In May 2013, when I (Kathryn) read the *New York Times* article "Some of My Best Friends Are Germs" by Michael Pollan, a brand-new world, quite literally, revealed itself to me: the human microbiome, our unique microbial ecosystem, comprising about 100 trillion bacteria that reside in, and on, all of us. Scientists have discovered that these elaborate communities of microbes regulate nearly every function in our bodies. They help us digest food and synthesize nutrients, and regulate our immune system, brain function, and emotions. Perhaps most astounding is the fact that these critters outnumber our human cells 10 to 1. This "second genome," as researchers are calling it, may have more of an impact on our overall health than the genes we inherited from our parents. This changed everything we thought we understood about human health and our relationship to the microbial world. If we are 10 percent human and 90 percent bacteria, has the war on bacteria been a war we've waged on ourselves? It seems so. In Pollan's *Times* article, he points out that "Such a paradigm shift comes not a moment too soon, because as a civilization, we've just spent the better part of a century doing our unwitting best to wreck the human-associated microbiota with a multifronted war on bacteria and a diet notably detrimental to its well-being."

Microbiome science is opening up not only a new way to think about our health, but also about all living systems. And after one hundred years of war on ourselves and the planet, maybe it's time to call a truce and rethink our relationship with nature. The Western gut seems like a good place to start.

The Cultured Gut

"Science is gradually confirming what traditional cultures always somehow just knew: that fermented foods are special foods, able to nourish us deeply and help keep us healthy."

—SANDOR ELLIX KATZ

No one can say exactly what an ideal gut microbiome looks like yet, but extensive, worldwide research is starting to provide clues. American Gut Project, cofounded by Jeff Leach and Rob Knight of Knight Labs, was a crowd-sourced, citizen science project that collected, sequenced, and compared microbiome samples from 2012 to 2019. Their work has shown that gut microbe diversity in Western populations is substantially less diverse than that of hunter-gatherer tribes in Africa and South America, who are more susceptible to infectious diseases but have almost none of our modern diseases such as diabetes, autism, arthritis, heart disease, or anything like our recent epidemic of autoimmune diseases. This phenomenon has led researchers to coin the term "The Impoverished Western Gut."

Researchers speculate that up to 90 percent of all diseases can be traced in some way back to the gut, and it appears that our guts may have a bigger problem than a lack of diversity—we may have "leaky guts." Processed foods, overuse of antibiotics in both humans and animals, rampant pesticide use, chlorinated water, and antibacterial soaps all contribute to this increasingly common condition. The lining of the intestines forms a barrier between the contents of the intestines and the rest of the body. If that lining for some reason becomes damaged, then toxins, antigens, and bacteria from the intestines can leak out into the bloodstream. This can cause the immune system to think the body is under attack, which sets in motion a counterattack that causes inflammation in the body. This in turn can cause anything from temporary discomfort to serious health issues. Chronic, low levels of inflammation have been linked to food sensitivities, allergies, nutrient malabsorption, inflammatory skin conditions, inflammatory bowel diseases, autoimmune diseases, and mood disorders.

SO WHAT'S A GUT TO DO?

An astonishing body of peer-reviewed research suggests that diets high in fiber and foods rich in the probiotics found in live-culture foods can help increase gut diversity. According to Dr. David Perlmutter, in his book *The Brain Maker*, "research shows that significant changes in the array of gut bacteria can happen in as little as 6 days." Like many doctors in recent years, Dr. Perlmutter recommends fermented, live-culture foods as part of his protocol for healing the gut.

Although bacteria, like *Lactobacilli*, found in live-culture foods are largely thought to be transient, they appear to help "nudge intestinal cells" to produce a protein that helps to seal the tight junctions in the gut lining, according to Justin and Erica Sonnenburg, microbiome research-ers at the Sonnenburg Lab at Stanford and authors of *The Good Gut*. The Sonnenburgs suggest that probiotic bacteria are like "UN peacekeepers, helping to enforce borders and deter aggressive forces." If human health is intrinsically related to increasing microbial diversity and healing the gut lining, then it would appear that including live-culture foods and drinks in your diet may be an excellent strategy for increasing overall well-being.

The benefits of fermentation go well beyond the production of probiotic bacteria. The process can make nutrients more available, remove toxins, and in some cases even generate new micronutrients not found in the raw ingredients. Fermented soy products such as tempeh, miso, and natto all employ microbes to convert hard-to-digest proteins into more digest-ible amino acids. Certain strains of lactic acid bacteria can also produce B vitamins, including vitamin B_{12}, according to an article published in the *Journal of Applied Microbiology* in December 2011. And fermenting cabbage into sauerkraut facilitates the breakdown of phytonutrients into cancer-fighting compounds called isothiocyanates and indole-3-carbinol.

The health benefits of including live cultures in your diet seem to be well supported by a growing body of research, but we are not health experts and are certainly not suggesting that fermented foods and bever-ages are a panacea for all health issues. Human bodies are complex, and nutrition is notoriously difficult to study because we are all so different. If live-culture foods are new for you, it may take some time for your body to adapt to the new microbes, especially if your gut microbiota is out of whack or limited in terms of diversity. Listen to your body as you try each new ferment, and know that gas is a normal part of the process and will lessen as your gut shifts to a healthier, more balanced state. Once there,

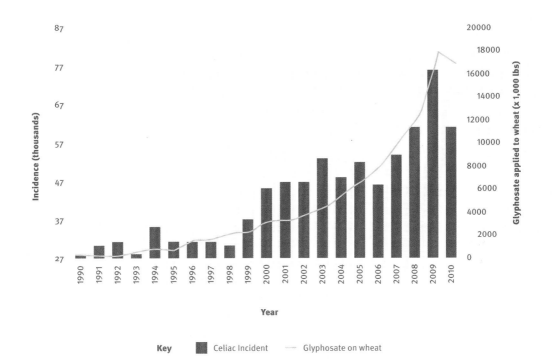

Key � Celiac Incident ── Glyphosate on wheat

THE ORGANIC CONNECTION

Glyphosate, the active ingredient found in the herbicide Roundup, is thought to be a particularly bad actor when it comes to gut permeability. In the intestines, glyphosate is a profound zonulin stimulator, which damages the epithelial "tight junction" tissue on contact, weakening the barriers that protect us on the inside from the outside. Interestingly, the protein gliadin, found in gluten, also stimulates the release of zonulin. The above graph shows an astounding correlation between the increased use of glyphosate on wheat crops (to help the wheat lay down better for the swather) starting in 1992 and celiac disease diagnoses.

Scientists are quick to point out that correlation is not causation and more research is needed, but the connection is compelling and certainly would explain why, after eating grains for thousands of years, many of us have all of a sudden become gluten intolerant. It seems that now more than ever, buying organic food—or, as your grandparents called it, "food"—is an important step in maintaining a healthy gut.

Hospital discharge diagnosis (any) of celiac disease ICD-9 579 and glyphosate applications to wheat (R=0.9759, p≤1.862e-06). Sources: USDA:NASS; CDC. (Figure courtesy of Nancy Swanson).

One of the most common and iconic vegetable ferments in the Western world is sauerkraut (fermented cabbage). Equally as ubiquitous in Korean culture and much of the East is the delicious and effervescent cabbage ferment known as kimchi. In fact, fermented cabbage was most likely the first lacto-fermented vegetable, and for good reason. Cabbage leaves are naturally covered in lactic acid bacteria, and are also full of sugars in the form of carbohydrates that are easily digested by bacteria. This makes cabbage a relatively easy vegetable to ferment, and a good entry point for beginners to the world of fermented food. Let's examine the lacto-fermentation process through the fermentation of sauerkraut on a microbial level and find out what's happening inside the crock.

Let's say you're making a batch of kraut. You shred a couple of heads of cabbage, massage them with salt at a measured rate, and pack the cabbage into a jar or crock, submerging it below the brine formed naturally by the liquid in the cabbage. Remember all those naturally present bacteria and yeasts? As soon as the cabbage is shredded, its sugars are exposed to the organisms present on the cabbage leaves, as well as the organisms present in the air, and they all begin to compete to eat those sugars at a rapid rate. With kraut, or any other lacto-fermented vegetable, you are trying to set the right circumstances for the lactic acid bacteria to thrive and outcompete the other microorganisms, allowing them to proliferate and acidify the ferment. The main way we do this is through the use of salt and temperature. By temporarily shifting the advantage to the halophilic (salt-tolerant) lactic acid bacteria, we are giving them an edge, just long enough for them to take hold and outcompete the other microorganisms. By fermenting at lower temperatures, we are also advancing the bacterial cause, as yeasts thrive in warmer conditions.

Once the stage is set and the crock is closed, the lactic acid bacteria begin to work their magic. First, a species of bacteria called *Leuconostoc mesenteroides* asserts its influence and begins transforming the ferment by producing acids and lowering the pH of the ferment. This first phase, commonly referred to as the heterolactic or gaseous phase, is characterized by the dominance of this species of lactic acid bacteria. *Leuconostoc* is a heterofermentative bacterium, meaning it produces more than one by-product. As it digests the sugars from the cabbage, it produces mostly lactic acid and minor amounts of acetic acid (vinegar), carbon dioxide, and alcohol as by-products (there are also other by-products produced but these are the primary ones). As the *Leuconostoc* proliferates, it produces lactic acid in abundance and alters the environment of the kraut, making it more acidic and inhibiting the growth of other yeasts and bacteria. *Leuconostoc* are the flavor-building bacteria. You want these heterofermentative bacteria to dominate the early stages of the fermentation. Lower temperatures and lower salt content are both favorable to *Leuconostoc*, whereas higher temperatures and higher salt levels will favor the highly acid-tolerant *Lactobacillus* species.

This is an important distinction to note for home fermenters, because if you ferment at too high a temperature or with too much salt, *Lactobacillus* will dominate from the beginning, producing a singularly sour ferment. The other important note to mention for the home fermenter is that you can gauge what phase of fermentation your jars or crocks are undergoing based on whether gas (carbon dioxide, or CO_2) is being produced. The production of gas assists in making the environment even more anaerobic, and thus favors the anaerobic organisms.

The *Leuconostoc* species are not as acid tolerant as other strains of lactic acid bacteria, so as the ferment gets more acidic, the *Leuconostoc* population dwindles. Much like the successive plants that colonize a disturbed forest, the initial bacterial species come in and alter the environment, making it more hospitable for the next successive wave of species to come in and occupy a different biological niche. After five to seven days, with the acidification under way, the microbial makeup of the ferment shifts and the acid-loving strains of bacteria, *Lactobacillus brevis* and *Lactobacillus plantarum*, begin to assert more influence over the ferment. We have now entered the second stage of fermentation, commonly referred to as the homolactic or nongaseous phase. These acid lovers are considered homofermentative bacteria, meaning they only produce one by-product: lactic acid (and lots of it!). They continue digesting the cabbage sugars and contributing to acidification, making it virtually impossible for any other organisms to live in the ferment. Other strains of *Lactobacillus* are commonly present during this stage, as well as other lactic acid bacteria such as *Pediococcus*. The acidification continues until the transformation is complete between twenty-one to twenty-eight days, producing a crunchy, tangy, and sour jar of goodness that will keep for years if refrigerated. At this point, if the fermentation is successful, the acidity will reach 1.6 percent and the pH will have dropped below 4.0, rendering the ferment acidic enough to be both well preserved and deemed "food-safe." The last bacteria standing is always *Lactobacillus plantarum*, which is the only species able to live in such an acidic environment. This is typically when the ferment would be moved into refrigeration. If left to ferment

SON-MAT

In Korea, if someone is a good cook, it is said that they possess *son-mat*, or good "hand taste." Traditionally, this compliment refers to a culinary talent, passed down through generations. If one is born with this quality, it is said that they have inherited a "great fortune." For many Koreans, the term also conjures the warmth and love a mother expresses in her cooking.

Jiwon Woo, artist, biodesigner, and researcher, conducted an award-winning study called "Mother's Hand Taste (Son-mat)" in 2017 at Utrecht University in the Netherlands.[1] Woo's project questioned if hand microbiomes influenced the process of fermentation and the taste of fermented food. She provided a recipe and the ingredients for *makgeolli*, a fermented rice wine, to twelve study participants spanning three generations, seven households, and four countries. She discovered that three of the four families possessed very similar hand microbes, regardless of their geographical location. How fascinating that this ancient term holds so much wisdom.

The study reminded Kathryn of the women she met in a small village outside Ollantaytambo in Peru who chewed corn into a mash that was then boiled and fermented into a delicious drink called *chicha*. A prerequisite for the job was a mouthful of saliva that contained an enzyme called ptyalin. Not everyone has this enzyme, but more women than men have it, and some possess a special version of it. One woman in the village was given special status and was revered for her particularly delicious *chicha*.

Perhaps that crock of sauerkraut on your kitchen counter is much more than just cabbage and salt. Within its walls lie generations of your family's unique microbial signature—a true family heirloom. Now *that's* something to celebrate!

1 Jiwon Woo, "Mother's Hand Taste (Son-mat)," www.woojiwon.com/mht-bad.

further, the pH will continue to drop to between 3.4 to 3.6 or even lower, resulting in a very sour kraut.

There are a multitude of factors at play every time you make a batch of lacto-fermented kraut (or any other lacto-ferment, for that matter). Everything contributes to and determines the final outcome of the ferment. The most crucial—but also most controllable—factors are the amount of salt used, temperature of the fermentation space, and time allowed for fermentation. Other contributing factors include the freshness of ingredients, the temperature of the produce (you want produce as close to the fermentation temperature as possible), the season, the atmospheric conditions of the day, the atmospheric conditions in your kitchen, the growing practices of the farmer, the post-harvest handling, your handling of the produce, the cleanliness of your kitchen and utensils and fermentation vessels, how long it takes you to get the ferment salted and submerged under the brine after you've sliced it . . . and let's not forget the microbes that you add to the ferment from your hands (see sidebar, opposite). Some people even take it as far as to ferment with the cycles of the moon! (We've made kraut on full moons, new moons, and everywhere in between, and have yet to notice a difference.) Another contributing factor is the cultural context from whence the ferment is made. Nearly every culture on the planet uses this ancient practice (or did at one time), but each place and people have their own methods, practices, and bacteria, or microbial terroir, all of which contribute to this global fabric of different flavors we call fermentation.

As you can see, many factors make up the microbial culture of a crock of sauerkraut. By managing those factors over which we do have control, such as salt and temperature, we are giving our ferments the best possible chance for success. We encourage you to pay close attention to the produce you buy for your ferments—ask the producers at your local farmers' market about their growing practices and when the produce was harvested (the fresher, the better). Hopefully the next time you pick up a jar of kraut, you will see deeper into the realm of the unseen little microbes responsible for making that sour and tangy ferment.

ALCOHOL FERMENTATION

Let us start by saying that alcohol is quite easy to make. Humans have been making hooch for thousands of years, and for one very good reason: it alters our consciousness. In nature, not many substances have the power to alter minds, and the ones that do are highly revered and coveted. The pursuit of this mind-altering buzz has built entire empires, is likely responsible for the advent of settled agriculture, and has changed the course of human history.

While making alcohol is quite simple, making really good alcohol is something else altogether. The fermentation science is very complicated, and each type of alcohol—wine, beer, mead, cider—has its own very different requirements, processes, and fermentations. For this reason, in this section we will be discussing the alcohol fermentation in a broad sense, as there are commonalities with all the previously mentioned alcohol ferments. For example, wine fermentation is very complicated at the commercial level, with all kinds of processes and additions, but you can make very tasty wine by simply crushing grapes and allowing the native microbes to ferment the sugars into alcohol. You don't need to be an expert or a microbiologist to make tasty homemade wine, beer, or mead, but having a basic understanding of the science behind the process will give you a better chance for success.

The catalyst for alcohol fermentation is yeast, and the yeast specifically responsible for all these fermented beverages is *Saccharomyces cerevisiae*. This species is widely used by humans for alcohol and bread fermentation, and within this species there are literally hundreds of different strains for the home brewer to choose from (see page 64 for yeast strains, starter cultures, and wild yeast traps).

It should be noted that while the alcohol fermentation will benefit from having some oxygen present in the initial phase, in the form of dissolved oxygen in the must (the liquid mixture prior to fermentation), the process should otherwise be carried out anaerobically in a sealed carboy. It could be said that the art of making alcohol is the art of *not* making vinegar. *Acetobacter* (the bacteria responsible for producing vinegar) is essentially everywhere: in the air, on the skins of fruit, and, if you use raw vinegar in your kitchen, most definitely there. If this bacteria infiltrates your hooch, it will turn it into vinegar. Vinegar is easy to make for this reason, whereas alcohol requires more care and vigilance.

Okay, now that you've been warned about the perils of *Acetobacter*, let's begin. Alcohol fermentation has three main phases:

1. The lag or adaptation phase
2. The primary fermentation phase
3. The secondary fermentation or conditioning phase

In an optimal fermentation where the yeast population is significant, the nutrition is adequate, and the sugar content and temperature are within the yeast's optimal range, the yeast should be able to move through all these stages in two to three weeks.

The exact ingredients and quantities will vary by type of beverage, but generally speaking, alcohol fermentation begins as soon as a sugar source is combined with water, creating what is called the must (an unfermented water and sugar solution), and the must is then exposed to the catalyst for the yeast fermentation, *Saccharomyces*, which is either added or naturally present in the must.

The *lag phase*, also called the *adaption phase* is essentially the period where the yeasts are acclimating to their new environment (temperature, nutrients, pH, and sugar level) and preparing for reproduction by

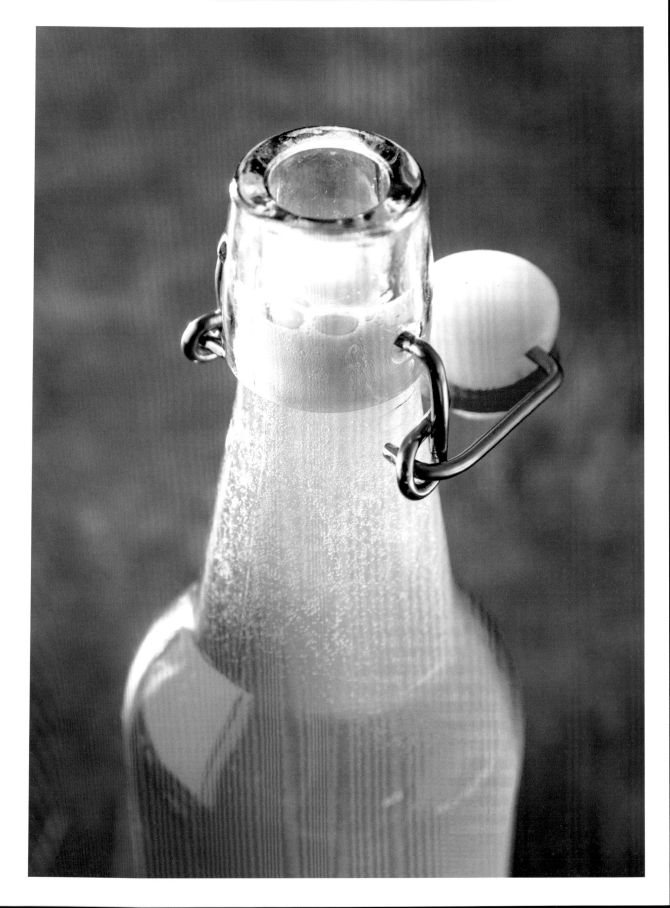

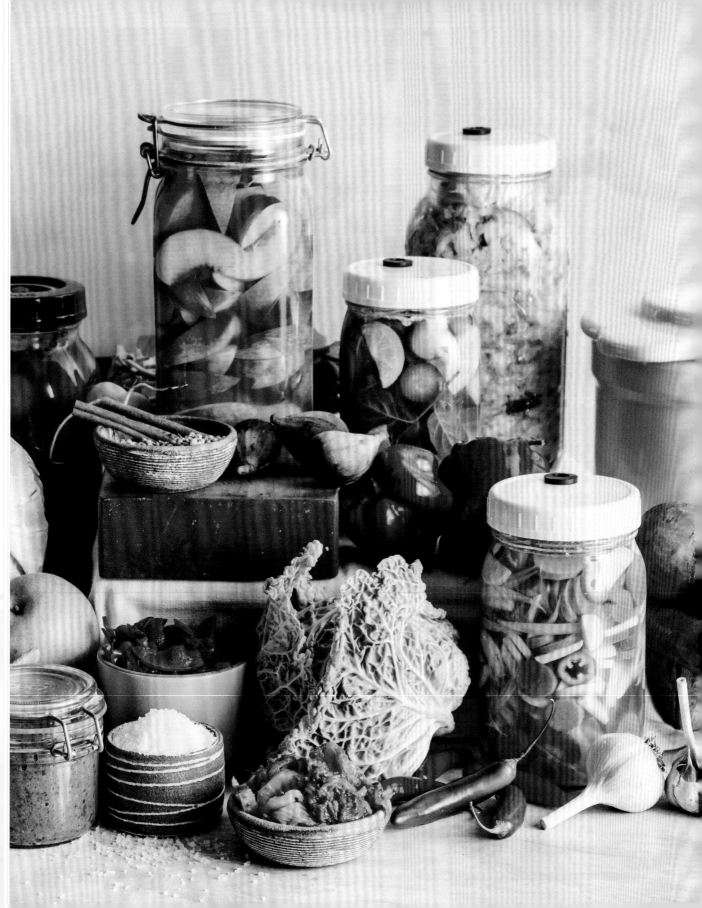

Fermentation 101

This section guides you through the myriad of possibilities and offers detailed descriptions to help you in choosing the right equipment and ingredients for your home ferments, as well as illustrating the upsides and pitfalls that are possible with each method. We'll run through the spectrum of options for fermentation vessels, specialized fermentation lids for lactic acid bacteria (LAB) ferments (including DIY options), all the necessary brewing equipment needed to make alcohol, and some vital ingredients, and also offer troubleshooting advice to assist you if and when things go awry.

Fermentation Equipment

Before you get started, it's important that you have some understanding of the basic equipment you'll need for your fermentation projects. Before starting a recipe or heading out to buy ingredients, check the recipe's Equipment list to ensure that you have the tools you'll need to complete the process. The Resources section on page 348 details where you can purchase the fermentation equipment we describe in the following pages.

Whatever vessel or sealing method you decide on, just know that there are bound to be successes and failures, and take solace in the fact that fermentation is on some levels under our control and on other levels completely out of our hands. At the end of the day, we are relying on the microbes to do most of the work, and much of what happens is up to them—all we can do is try to give the desired organisms the edge they need to flourish.

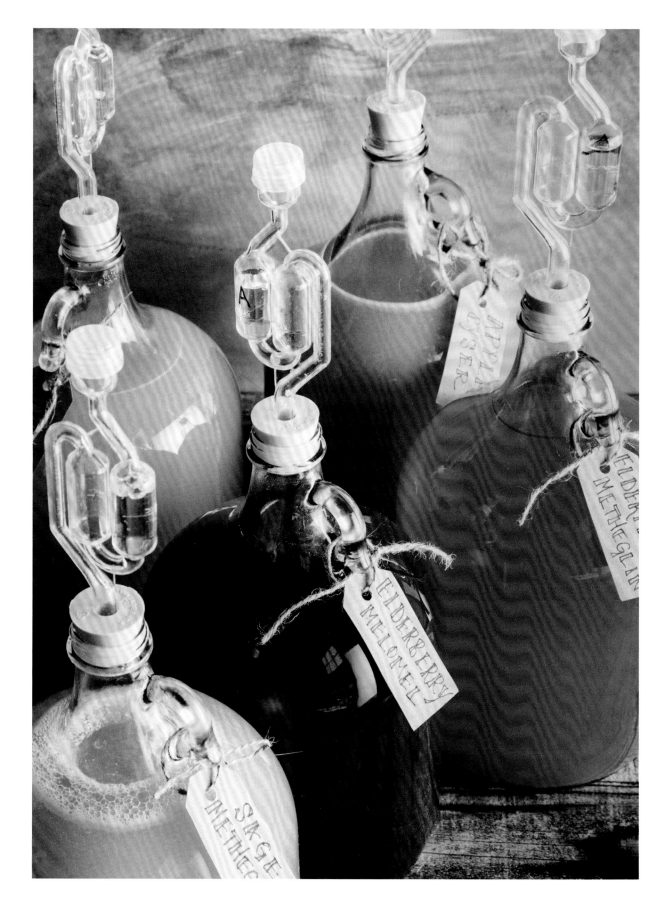

JARS AND FERMENTATION LIDS

For most of the recipes in this book, all you need is a 1-quart or ½-gallon wide-mouth glass canning jar and a lid fitted with an airlock. The main purpose of the fermentation vessel is to maintain an anaerobic (oxygen-less) environment while still allowing gas to escape (CO_2), a by-product of microbial metabolism of the lactic acid fermentation. While crocks are a great piece of equipment for fermentation, they are expensive, and so canning jars fitted with a specialized fermentation lid are really the way to go. Since the jar system is inexpensive, it is a great way to get started and try your hand at fermentation without spending too much money upfront. The other advantage of a jar system, and why we still choose this system for our ferments, is that it allows the home fermenter to make lots of ferments cheaply and effectively.

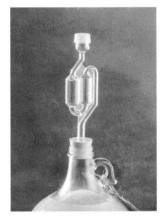

DIY Airlock Lid

Specialized fermentation lids can be expensive (some running as high as $30 per lid), especially if you are doing a lot of fermenting, so I (Shane) prefer to make my own. The advantages of this system are that it's inexpensive, easy to make yourself, and easy to use, and you can use the same lid system on different size jars. The downside is that with all the components and points of seal, you can have a breach somewhere in the system, which could result in yeast and/or mold issues.

The number-one reason I prefer a simple lid fitted with an airlock is that you can actually see the fermentation action occurring through the percolation of water through the airlock. Having an accurate visual cue will give you a better understanding of what's happening inside the jar. When you set a ferment in motion, it is quite satisfying, and almost a relief, to see the bubbles and hear the *blurp, blurp* of the airlock bubbling away. This sound tells you that the bacteria or yeasts are strong and present, and that the heterofermentative stage of the LAB fermentation process (when gas and other by-products are being produced) is under way. This gives you a better understanding of which stage of the fermentation process your ferment is undergoing.

Specialized Lids

For those who have no interest in making their own lids and just want to purchase a system, there are many options available. Karla Delong, the fabulous fermentista from Mountain Feed & Farm Supply and one of the most experienced home fermenters we know, has probably tested just

DIY AIRLOCK SYSTEM #1

This setup is very close to the Perfect Pickler system (see page 44), which costs about $13 per kit. The DIY components can be purchased online for about $4.30 per system ($6.50 if using a ½-gallon jar). Most of the components come in packs of three or five, and ½-gallon jars come in cases of six, so essentially, you could make five or six systems for the price of two Perfect Picklers.

Wide-mouth gasket

Wide-mouth white plastic lid

⅜-inch rubber grommet

Airlock

Wide-mouth glass jar

1. Using a ½-inch drill bit, drill a hole into the center of the lid.
2. Insert the grommet. (I had to learn the hard way that if you drill a ⅜-inch hole, it will be too small for a ⅜-inch grommet—grommets are sized by their inner dimension, and the outer dimension is slightly larger.)
3. Insert the airlock into the grommet.
4. Prepare your ferment in the jar. Place the gasket inside the lid, screw on the lid, and you're ready to go! It's that simple.

Note: If you're not comfortable drilling a hole into the plastic lids, you can purchase just the predrilled lids with the grommet from Perfect Pickler for only $3.95. You will still need to purchase airlocks and gaskets for the lid.

DIY AIRLOCK SYSTEM #2

Another DIY lid system forgoes the airlock altogether and instead utilizes plastic tubing running from the lid into a basin filled with water. This method requires less components than the one previously mentioned, and allows the home fermenter to run multiple ferments into the same basin filled with water. To make, simply drill a hole in a wide-mouth plastic lid, insert a grommet as directed above, then cut and insert about a 3-feet-long piece of ⅜-inch food-grade silicone or plastic tubing (available at brewing supply stores or online) into the grommet and run that tube into a bowl, cup, or pitcher of water. Prepare your ferment in the jar, place a wide-mouth gasket inside the lid, and screw on the lid. The nice thing about this system is that you avoid the cost of buying airlocks. If you make the tube long enough and position the vessel of water above the ferment (say, on a shelf above it), you can avoid some of the messy "boilovers" that you might have with an airlock.

about every newfangled fermentation contraption on the market, and was kind enough to share her review of the best fermentation lids: "The **Perfect Pickler** works great, as long as the gaskets are sound. The best lid for short-term ferments is **Kraut Source**, and the best for long term is the **Ferment'n** system. The easiest to use is the **Pickle Pipe**, but take caution, as the lid can fail with large swings in temperature."

Lid Safety

When using any of the aforementioned lids for fermentation, if you have a breach in one of the seals, you can have issues with yeast and/or mold growing on the surface of the ferment. Checking the seals during the first few days of fermentation is important to ensure that you don't have any breaches. Once gases are being produced (this is usually quite evident after two to three days of fermentation), fill a spray bottle with some soapy water and spray around the lid as well as around all seals and the base of the airlock. The soapy water will show you if you have any breaches, as little bubbles will form where gas is being expelled. You only want air to escape through the airlock or designated hole. If gas is escaping through any other seal, that means oxygen is getting in, too, and bringing all kinds of contaminative microbes with it. This is more important with longer ferments such as kraut or pepper mash.

CROCKS

If you're just getting started with home fermenting, we highly recommend that you buy some of the aforementioned ½-gallon jars and fermentation lids, and avoid spending a bunch of money until you know it is something that you will be doing regularly. But if you *really* get into fermenting or want to make larger batches, then crocks are an excellent way to go. A crock

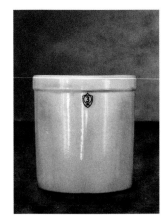

is a stoneware pot, usually ceramic or clay, designed specifically for fermentation. They are available in two main categories—water sealed and open top—and come in many different sizes, shapes, and styles. Which you choose really depends on what you are fermenting. Typically, 1- and 2-gallon crocks are excellent options for most home fermenters, as these volumes should accommodate most of your desired batch sizes. If you are making open-top alcohol ferments, you will probably want a larger crock.

Look to your local community for beautiful handmade crocks. Often you can find a unique crock made by a local artisan. Just be sure that if you buy a water-sealed crock from an artist, the moat is deep enough and shaped properly to accommodate the water. We bought a beautiful handmade ceramic crock from a local artisan, but unfortunately the moat was so shallow and misshapen that the water was lost to evaporation and spillage, requiring daily attention and essentially rendering the crock useless for anything other than open-top fermentation.

Water-Sealed Crocks

If you want a crock for making lacto-fermented fruits and vegetables, we advise using a water-sealed crock. The defining feature with water-sealed crocks is that they have a moat around the top rim where the lid sits; the moat is filled with water and creates a water-locked seal when the lid is in place. Gases produced through the fermentation process will bubble up through the water and can escape beneath the lid, but oxygen can't penetrate the seal. Polish-made crocks are water-sealed and are made of highly enriched vitrified clay, which is one of the strongest building materials for clay pottery and ceramics. Harsch Gärtopf fermenting crocks from Germany are another excellent water-sealed option. Ohio Stoneware, the most widely available American producer, makes a really beautiful water-sealed crock, though it is only available in a 3-gallon size. We have fermented in this crock for many years, and have found that while the larger size is a bit too big for the batch sizes of most ferments in the home kitchen, it is perfect for making cucumber pickles, which are so seasonal that its often necessary to make larger batches during the height of the cucumber season.

There are many upsides to using water-sealed crocks:

➤ They require very little attention to keep your ferments anaerobic (topping off the water in the moat occasionally is all that's needed).

- You won't have to deal with messy "boilovers" resulting from brine escaping through lids or airlocks, which can cause quite a smelly mess if left unattended.
- They are easy to clean, and you don't have to deal with cleaning and sanitizing a number of small components as with an airlock system.

The downsides are few—mainly the expense—but larger crocks are heavy and may be difficult for some people to handle. If you do decide to purchase a water-sealed crock, make sure it comes with glass or ceramic weights. Most do, but some companies will make you purchase weights and lids separately. The weights are placed inside the crock, on top of the ferment, to keep all the solids submerged under the brine.

Open-Top Crocks

Open-top crocks can be utilized for aerobic ferments that do not require the anaerobic environment facilitated by a lid with a water moat. If you will be using a crock solely for SCOBY or vinegar fermentation, which can all be made aerobically (with exposure to oxygen), then you can go with the open-top crock option. These crocks are just a simple vessel with no lid, weights, or water moat, and are typically much less expensive than water-sealed crocks. Lids and weights can usually be purchased separately for these crocks, and people do use the open-top crock for anaerobic ferments such as pickles and kraut, but we highly recommend that you don't, as the aerobic environment will likely lead to yeast and/or mold contamination in the upper reaches of the ferment. These crocks are really much better suited for aerobic ferments, and a lid and weights are unnecessary for this process. Cheesecloth or cotton fabric can be used to cover the top and keep insects out while allowing oxygen to enter the crock. If you are using a crock solely for the fermentation of kombucha, then we highly recommend that you buy a 1-gallon glass jar with a spigot. These glass jars with spigots allow you to taste the fermenting kombucha without disturbing the mother floating on top.

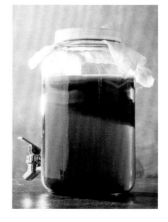

Open-top crocks can also be utilized for the first three to four days of alcohol fermentation. This helps infuse oxygen into the must, which the yeast uses during the respiratory phase. The open-top crock is also an excellent option for fermenting alcohol with the addition of fruit and/or herbs in the primary fermentation. For instance, in red wine production, the primary fermentation of the must is carried out in an open-top fermentation vessel with the skins, seeds, and stems all combined in the vessel, all

ONGGI POTS

Maybe it's because our ancient ancestors fermented in earthenware pots, or perhaps because it is a beautiful natural material in an age of plastic, but there is just something about using an elemental earthenware crock that seems right. Along this line, *onggi* pots, the traditional earthenware crocks used in Korea to ferment kimchi, actually allow the ferment inside to "breathe." Onggi pots have a microporous structure to the clay, which allows gases to escape while not permitting oxygen to enter. They are traditionally buried in the earth, which keeps the ferment at a stable temperature, which just happens to be an excellent temperature for kimchi fermentation. I think Michael Pollan eloquently captures the essence of fermenting in earthenware crocks in his book *Cooked*: "The earthenware crock is a good reminder that every ferment is food and drink stolen, or borrowed, from the earth, by temporarily diverting its microbial-gravitational pull to our own ends." Though you probably won't be fermenting in onggi pots buried in the earth, using earthenware crocks for fermentation reconnects us to our ancestral roots deep in the earth, and serves as a beautiful reminder of the temporary nature of all things.

of which contribute flavorful elements to the sensory profile of the finished wine. When you ferment the must with fruit or plant material in an open-top crock, using the fermentation process along with time to extract flavor from the fruit and/or herbs, this process infuses aromatic compounds into the must and enhances the flavor of the finished beverage. This method allows the home fermenter to easily infuse flavor and tannins into the must, while allowing for ease of straining and transferring of the liquid must, as well as making it easy to clean the vessel once the must has been racked into a sealed carboy. If you tried to ferment a batch of wine with the fruit in a sealed carboy, it would be very difficult to strain the must off the fruit and very difficult to clean afterwards. Because kombucha, vinegar, and even the primary fermentation of alcohol can all be produced aerobically, an open-top crock is really the way to go, as it is a cheap and versatile piece of fermentation equipment that can be effectively used for all the aforementioned ferments, as well as any other anaerobic ferment.

BUCKETS AND WATER BAGS

Another DIY system that works really well, especially for larger batches, is the water bag method. This method can be used very effectively to ferment in larger plastic containers, such as food-grade 5-gallon buckets, and is a cheap way to make large batches of a ferment without having to purchase a costly crock. For farmers and homesteaders who have large quantities of produce to preserve and not a lot of money to spend on their fermentation setup, this is by far the best method. To create a water bag seal, fill two or three small (1-quart) ziplock bags with water. Fill a large, wide-mouth vessel with your ferment, leaving the top quarter of the vessel empty to allow space for the water bags. Place a liner bag (such as a large ziplock freezer bag or another thick plastic bag) into the vessel, and place the water-filled smaller bags into the liner bag. This creates a seal that oxygen cannot penetrate, while allowing gas to escape. It also exerts downward pressure on the ferment to keep the solids submerged in the brine. This technique can also be used in large jars, but if you fill the jar too full with the ferment, there won't be enough room left to create a good seal with the water bags. Many people advocate using the water bag method in jars, but we typically don't advise it; there are better methods. Where this method does come in handy is when you don't have enough produce to fill your jar to the top. For instance, if you have a certain amount of a produce that you want to ferment, but not enough to fill the desired jar size, then using the water bag method is preferable to having a large amount of empty headspace, which often results in contamination from airborne organisms.

VACUUM-SEALED BAGS

In the summer of 2014, we were lucky enough to get a table at Noma, which at the time was ranked as the number one restaurant in the world. Not only is Noma unparalleled when it comes to Nordic cuisine, their team is doing some of the most interesting and provocative fermentation in the entire world. During the course of our meal, we ate a few dishes with a fermented mushroom sauce, and at dessert we were blissfully served porcini mushrooms (*Boletus edulis*, aka the king bolete) that had been fermented, dehydrated, and covered in dark chocolate and sea salt. After that transcendent lunch, knowing that we were fermentation geeks, they offered us a tour of their state-of-the-art fermentation lab, aptly dubbed "the Science Bunker." When we entered the Science Bunker, we were pleasantly surprised to see the source of all that umami goodness: porcinis, floating in a brine of their own juices, fermenting in vacuum-sealed bags. Voilà! A lightbulb went on and we have been employing this technique for LAB fermentation ever since. The vacuum-bag method is an effective and relatively inexpensive way to create an anaerobic environment for LAB fermentation.

There are several great things about fermenting in vacuum-sealed bags:

- You can see what is happening with the ferment through the clear plastic.
- You can see the gases being expressed, as the bag will bloat and expand when the LAB ferment is in the heterofermentative stage.
- You can very effectively make small-batch ferments.
- While the sealing machine is an upfront expense, the vacuum bags are quite inexpensive.

All that being said, the plastic waste is definitely not ideal for the conscientious consumer (the world is already choking on way too much plastic), so if you're weary of plastic in general, this is not the option for you. You can also encounter issues if you have a breach in the bags during fermentation, which can result in a briny mess. When employing this method, it is important to keep an eye on the bag as it bloats, and if necessary, cut one end off to release the built up gases, then reseal. The bags are pretty sturdy, and we have not personally had a bag explode as a result of the fermentation action, but we could imagine that an extremely active ferment could cause the bag to expand beyond its limits.

WEIGHTS

In many ferments, the solids will float to the top, being thrust upward by the force of the escaping CO_2. If your lid or seal is good, the CO_2 produced will create an environment in the headspace (the empty space between the top of the ferment and the top of the vessel) that makes it virtually impossible for other organisms to grow there. However, if your lid or seal has leaks, contamination is likely. To prevent this, fermenters use weights or other systems to keep the solids in the ferment submerged beneath the brine.

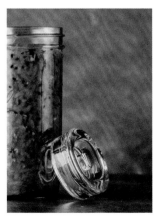

We have found that **glass weights** are especially useful and fit nicely into standard and wide-mouth jars. The Easy Weight is a popular glass weight; it fits wide-mouth canning jars and has a built-in grooved handle for easy placement and removal. You can also buy plastic inserts, such as ViscoDisc Canning Buddies, which are significantly cheaper than glass weights but are most effective with ferments that have a lot of liquid. Through the course of writing this book, we have both become converts to glass weights, owing to the fact that they really do help achieve more consistent results, especially with longer ferments like krauts and pepper mashes.

A DIY trick we learned from Karla Delong is to buy **thin plastic cutting boards**, which are cheap, and then cut them into round disks that match the inner circumference of your vessel at its widest point. You can then bend them to fit into the mouth. Once inserted, the disk will expand and act as a wedge, keeping the solids below the brine. Punching a couple of holes into the disk allows the free flow of brine and gases, while keeping the solids submerged. This method is especially useful for ferments that contain brine, such as all the brined ferments and the sour tonic recipes in this book, as the vegetable pieces have a tendency to float, and the cutting board disk keeps the pieces safely submerged below the brine level.

And finally, a **cabbage leaf** or really any vegetable placed between the ferment and the lid can be used to push the solids below the brine, and can be used instead of purchased weights. Any root vegetable, for instance, can be cut into a round disk 1 to 2 inches thick and placed on top of a ferment instead of a weight.

KRAUT TAMPER

A tamper is any long, thin device with one flat end that is used to pack down, or "tamp" down, a ferment as you are putting it into your vessel. Packing your dry-salted ferments down (brined ferments don't need tamping down) is an important step that forces out air pockets and helps to fully submerge the solids under the naturally produced brine. If you can easily fit your hand into a wide-mouth canning jar, then a kraut tamper is unnecessary, as a hand does the job of tamping down even more efficiently. However, if you have large hands and can't easily fit them into a wide-mouth canning jar, then this device is most welcome and really helps the process. You can purchase wooden kraut tampers online, available through most websites that sell fermentation equipment, or you can use the blunt end of any piece of kitchen equipment that you own that fits into the jar, such as the tamper tool that comes with most blenders or a meat tenderizer.

CANNING FUNNEL

A canning funnel is a cheap and widely available piece of equipment that aids in the process of transferring a ferment, after mixing, from the bowl to the fermentation vessel. Because the mouth of canning jars is so small, this process can be quite messy and so the canning funnel, with its wide top tapering down to fit inside wide-mouth canning jars, can really help to limit spillage.

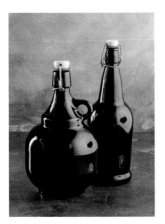

BREWING EQUIPMENT

You can go crazy buying brewing equipment, as there is essentially a piece of equipment available for every aspect of the process. While some of these technologies are worthwhile and make the task of brewing much easier, many are unnecessary for the home brewer. For the alcohol ferments in this book, we have chosen to present you with the most streamlined and cost-effective methods, using as little equipment as possible, and will leave it up to you to decide whether you need any other specialized equipment.

The main tools you need for brewing are a carboy, a bung, an airlock, a siphon, and a hydrometer. All these tools are inexpensive and widely available. Unlike fermentation lids and seals, which come in many different styles, these basic brewing tools are pretty much standard. Brewing supply stores are great resources for equipment and often have brewing experts on staff who can be very helpful in answering your fermentation and equipment questions. If you really get into brewing your own booze, I highly recommend seeking out your local brewing supply store and talking to the experts there.

Carboys are glass or plastic jugs fitted with a bung and an airlock, and are used solely for the brewing of fermented beverages, typically alcohol. They can be used for fermentation from start to finish, or a ferment that has finished its first stage in an open-top crock or container can be racked into an airlock-sealed carboy to finish fermenting. Carboys come in different sizes, but 1, 3, 5, or 6 gallons are commonly available. All the alcohol recipes in this book are made in 1-gallon batches, for a few reasons:

- ▸ It is easier to scale up from 1 gallon to larger volumes than it is to scale down.
- ▸ If you lose a 1-gallon batch to a defect, or you don't really like the finished beverage, it's not as tragic as losing all the effort and ingredients you poured into a 5-gallon batch.
- ▸ Working in 1-gallon carboys allows more experimentation with different techniques and ingredients and will afford you more variety of finished drinks.
- ▸ Making a 3- or 5-gallon batch makes sense if you are pressing apples or another fruit and have lots of juice that you want to turn into cider, but other than that, 5 gallons can be just too much of a good thing.

- One-gallon carboys are easier to handle and move around, whereas full 5-gallon carboys are quite heavy and can be hard to manage.

If you find a recipe you really like and want to make a larger batch, you can easily scale up the 1-gallon recipe by multiplying the ingredients to fit whatever size vessel you choose.

To ferment in a carboy, you'll also need a **bung**, a slightly tapered round silicone or rubber stopper with a hole through the center that fits into the top of the carboy. Bungs come in many different sizes; 6.5 is the right size for a 1-gallon carboy. If you're using another size carboy, make sure you also buy the correct size bung.

Airlocks are a one-size-fits-all piece of equipment. They come in a few different styles, but the concept is the same for all of them: The airlock is filled with water to the designated fill line and is inserted into the bung. The water creates a natural seal that allows gas (CO_2) to escape while not permitting oxygen to enter the vessel. I prefer S-shaped airlocks because they have fewer parts to deal with, but a three-piece airlock can be disassembled for easier cleaning. They are both totally acceptable, and which you use really depends on your preference. When fermenting, keep an eye on the airlock to make sure it never runs dry, cleaning it and refilling with fresh water as needed, although this is only really an issue in very long ferments, like the two-month pepper mash ferments (see page 184).

A **siphon** is a plastic tube with a smaller plastic tube inside it, attached to a piece of flexible tubing, used for racking. A siphon is often used in conjunction with a **racking cane**, which is nothing more than a stick that keeps the siphon tube above the settled yeast in the fermentation vessel. Siphons are useful and cheap, and are widely available online or at your local brewing supply store. Racking with a siphon has quite a few advantages over simply pouring your brew into a bottle:

- Racking limits the exposure of the brew to oxygen, which can result in contamination from undesirable microbes, such as *Acetobacter*.
- It limits the oxidative effect from the liquid being exposed to oxygen, resulting in less vibrant colors.
- It is an efficient way to move liquid around and requires less manual effort to bottle your brew.
- It allows you to transfer your brew to bottles, while leaving the unwanted flocculated yeast behind.

A **wine thief** is another useful piece of equipment. It is a tube with a valve on the bottom that enables you to pull samples from your alcohol ferments while limiting exposure to oxygen. When fermenting alcohol, being able to pull a sample for both sensory evaluation and to measure specific gravity (see hydrometers, below) is important to help you gauge whether the ferment is ready for bottling. Wine thieves are cheap and widely available.

A **hydrometer** is an instrument for measuring the dissolved solids in a liquid, or more specifically, the amount of sugar dissolved in a solution. Hydrometers are cheap (about $10) and are a very useful tool for home fermenters. They look like a thermometer with a wider bottom, tapering to a thinner dimension at the top, and they come on a plastic cylinder that is used to hold the liquid you intend to measure. The most common measurement scale used on the hydrometer is called specific gravity. There are other scales on the device, such as Plato, Brix, and Balling, but they all essentially measure the same thing using different numbers, and for our purposes, all you need to know is how to use the specific gravity measurement. The amount of sugar present in the must prior to fermentation is referred to as the original gravity (OG), also commonly called starting gravity, and the amount of sugar present at the time of bottling is called the finished gravity (FG). Water at a temperature of 68°F has a specific gravity of 1.000. As you add sugar, the density of the liquid increases and raises the specific gravity. Measuring specific gravity in your alcohol ferments, both pre- and post-fermentation is important because:

- You can use the OG measurement to calculate what the potential alcohol in the finished beverage will be if the fermentation is successful
- If you know the OG and the FG, you can calculate what the actual alcohol content is in the finished beverage.
- You can use the OG and subsequent measurements to assess how the fermentation is progressing.
- You can compare the OG and FG to gauge when your beverage is ready for bottling.

It probably sounds much more complicated than it actually is in practice, so don't be intimidated. If you can use a thermometer, then you can use a hydrometer. The one variable that does affect all this is the temperature of the liquid at the time of measurement. There are multiple complicated formulas for calculating alcohol by volume (ABV), but I recommend that you

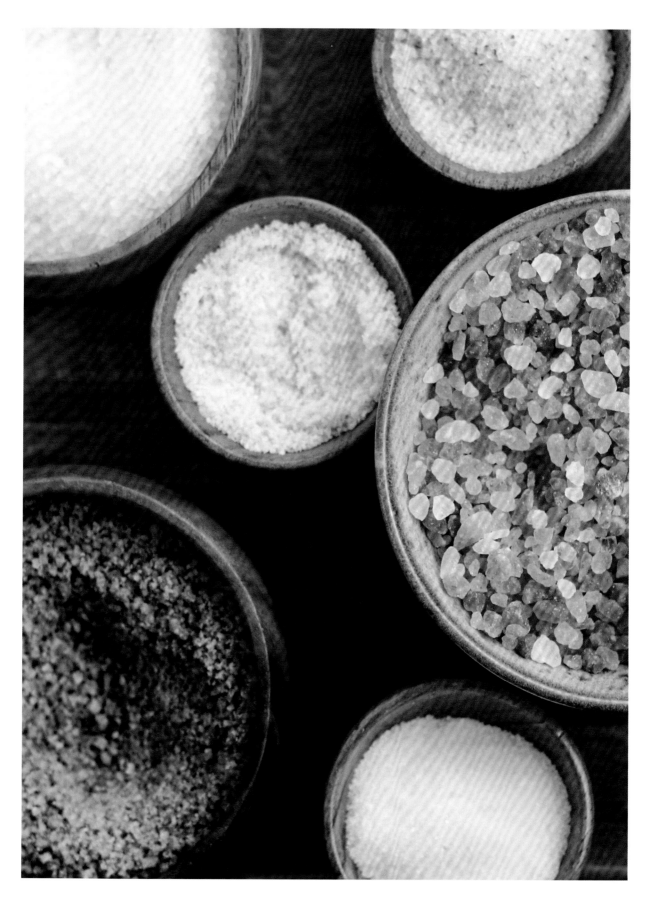

use one of the many online calculators available for this. Most of these calculators take into account the temperature, making it much easier than doing the math yourself.

KITCHEN SCALE

A kitchen scale is a worthwhile investment and is critical to achieving accurate fermentation. Every ardent home cook should have a digital kitchen scale, as they are inexpensive and very useful, especially for fermentation and baking. Many people experienced with fermenting choose to salt their ferments by taste, and once you have enough experience, you can, too. But when you're first starting out, it's better to be accurate. Even with all our experience, we still weigh out all our ingredients every time to achieve the most consistent results possible.

For the recipes in this book, it was our goal to give precise and accurate measurements, choosing weight over volume and metric over imperial measures (see page 76 for more on the measurements in this book). This stems partly from years of experience fermenting, knowing that accuracy is crucial, and also partly from frustration trying to follow inaccurate recipes calling for "1 carrot" or a "bunch of radishes," which makes it very difficult to get accurate salt percentages or to re-create a recipe successfully. The same is true of salt: different salts have different densities, so the percentages will vary depending on the salt you use. The only way to be completely accurate with your ingredients is to weigh them. With precise quantities of your ingredients going into your crock or jar, you can be assured of great success in your fermentation exploits. Do yourself a favor: if you don't have a kitchen scale, go buy one.

Ingredients

In this next section, we'll run you through some of the basic ingredients that are vital to fermentation, to ensure that you have the best ingredients available to produce beautiful ferments at home. We will shed light on salt types, varieties, and grain sizes, and the acceptable types of water to be used for your home ferments; offer some tips on produce as well as how to calculate waste and procure the proper quantities; and finally, we will run you through the different types of microbial starter cultures, including those available for purchase, as well as how to utilize LAB wild fermentation and how to make yeast traps to capture wild yeasts for your homemade hooch.

SALT, A PILLAR OF HUMANITY

Salt has become so commonplace, sitting neatly in little shakers on tables the world over, that we have all come to take it for granted. Such was not the case for our not-so-distant ancestors, for whom salt was a highly prized, extremely valuable commodity. Today, salt is in such abundance that we forget its bygone past, when the quest for salt built cities, defined the outcome of warfare, and was the catalyst for many of humanity's inventions and technologies. As Mark Kurlansky states in *Salt*, his provocative historical treatise on the subject:

> A number of the greatest public works ever conceived were motivated by the need to move salt. Salt has been in the forefront of the development of both chemistry and geology. Trade routes that have remained major thoroughfares were established, alliances built, empires secured, and revolutions provoked—all for something that fills the oceans, bubbles up from springs, forms crusts in lake beds, and thickly veins a large part of the earth's rock fairly close to the ace.

Salt is a catalyst for fermentation and preservation, forces that enabled humans to extend the shelf life of all manner of food and drink. With the advent of agriculture, for the first time in human history, we had large quantities of food that needed to be preserved. We also had livestock that required salt, both for the animals' health and to preserve their meat after slaughter. One could conjecture that without the preservative power of salt, human civilization could not have risen so quickly and ubiquitously to its place at the top of the food chain.

SALT

When we say "salt," we're talking about what we all commonly refer to as salt: sodium chloride (NaCl). Edible salt can be broken into two main categories: evaporated salt from the ocean or brine springs, and mined rock salt, both of which contain minerals of varying types in varying degrees and both of which we have used in ferments with great success. Within these categories, the home fermenter has many options to choose from, as any salt can be used for fermentation as long as it hasn't been highly processed and contains no additives.

So what kind of salt should you use? To a certain degree, this is a matter of preference, and is also contingent on what you have available near you. But we highly encourage you to find and use the most local salt you can. A local salt will add a unique element and contribute to the terroir of your home ferments. For some of you, this might not be realistic, as salt production is limited to coastal areas and areas with naturally occurring rock salt. But as with buying your produce, part of the intrigue of fermenting is looking to your local food shed, the geographic area between where your food is produced and consumed, for unique elements to add to your home ferments.

Kathryn and I (Shane) differ in our opinions about the best salt for fermenting. I prefer to work with unrefined sea salt and mineral salts, which are not highly processed and retain much of the mineral content from the ocean, brine spring, or mine where they were harvested. Though typically present in small quantities, these minerals will assist in the fermentation process and also make your finished product more nutritious. It should be noted that highly mineralized salts, while adding minerals to your ferment, do contain slightly less sodium chloride. This difference, though typically minuscule, will ultimately lower the salt content of your ferment by a fraction of a percent. This should not negatively affect the process, but it's something to consider. Mineral salts can also be unpredictable, as the differing mineral contents can have varying effects on the microbial communities in your crock. Salt that is high in calcium and magnesium will positively influence the crunch of your ferments, helping to strengthen the cell walls of the vegetables and limiting degradation of the pectic cell walls, which leads to softening. Kathryn prefers to work with a purer sea salt, with higher sodium chloride content and fewer minerals. She thinks these salts are more reliable and result in a cleaner flavor. It is true that unrefined salts vary widely in their mineral content and can have very different effects on the fermentation process. For commercial production, consistency is important, but the home fermenter is free to choose. We encourage you to play with different salts and see what works for you.

We used Sonoma sea salt (see page 58), a coarse-grain sea salt, to develop all the recipes in this book. We prefer a coarse-grain salt because the coarser grain helps break down the cell walls of plant materials, which is necessary for dry-salted ferments. For this reason, we specifically call for a coarse-grain salt in all the dry-salted recipes in the book. Some people prefer using finer salts because they dissolve more quickly into brine solutions, but we use hot water in our brined ferments, which dissolves coarse salt very easily, so the use of finer salt is unnecessary. That being said, there are numerous varieties of salt that you can use with great success so we did not specify salt grain size for any ferments containing brine—you can use either coarse or a finer grain size for brined ferments with equal success.

But let's start with one salt you should *not* use: **iodized salt**. Common table salt is typically iodized, meaning iodine has been added to it. This practice dates back to the 1920s, when, in collaboration with the government, salt manufacturers began adding iodine to counteract iodine deficiency in the American diet. Iodized table salt is highly refined, completely stripped of its mineral content, and combined with chemical anticaking agents, making it ill suited to your fermentation practices. Iodine can oxidize during the fermentation process and cause darkening or cloudiness in your lacto-ferments; it also has antimicrobial properties that could be unfavorable to the desired bacteria. For us, procuring fresh and beautiful ingredients is part of the fun, and if we're going to take so much care with our produce, why would we used a highly processed iodized salt when there are so many better options?

Sonoma sea salt is probably our favorite sea salt to work with—and as we mentioned, we used it to develop all the recipes in this book. When Kathryn set out to start Farmhouse Culture, she went on a quest to find the most local and sustainable salt available near our production location in Santa Cruz, California. She finally found Sonoma Pacific Sea Salt, an amazing local sea salt produced by SaltWorks. Since then, we've made literally millions of pounds of kraut with it, and we think it's a lovely salt for fermentation. The salt is harvested in Northern California from solar evaporation ponds drawn from the Pacific Ocean. It's available in multiple grain sizes, making it versatile for many different applications. It has no anticaking agents and is about as clean a salt as you can get.

Celtic sea salt is a lovely coarse-grain salt to ferment with. It is hand-harvested from pristine coastal regions in a process that utilizes the sun and the wind to evaporate the seawater into salt crystals. It is not highly refined and retains much of the mineral content from the sea. It contains seventy-four trace minerals and its gray tint comes from the clay in the evaporation ponds. Solar-evaporated sea salts like this one, depending on the process, typically retain most of their minerals.

Himalayan pink salt is a highly mineralized rock salt that is mined 5,000 feet below the Himalayas in Pakistan. It's an excellent choice for fermenting. It's hand harvested and sustainable, and contains over eighty-four minerals and trace elements, including calcium, magnesium, potassium, iron, and copper. The one downside is that Himalayan salt is just about as nonlocal as you can get, unless you are in Pakistan. It is, however, a lovely salt and has gained much notoriety and popularity due to its sustainability and health-enhancing minerals.

When I was homesteading, we had the loveliest well water on our property. This well water consistently produced some of the best kombucha, kefir, alcohol, and brined ferments that I have ever made, mostly due to the high mineral content of the water. Every well will have a different mineral makeup, which in turn will have varying effects on fermentation. You can have your well water tested for mineral content, which will tell you exactly which minerals are present. I am not an expert on well water, but I know that ours was high in calcium and manganese, and this produced very fine fermented foods and drinks. Water that is high in calcium and magnesium will positively affect the texture of fruit and vegetable ferments, because both help to reinforce cell-wall pectins.

—Shane

Pickling salt, highly refined pure sodium chloride marketed specifically for canning, preserving, and pickling, is an acceptable salt for fermentation. It has a finer grain, which helps it dissolve into brine solutions, but it's less desirable for dry-salted ferments. Ball and Morton make pickling salts, which may be available at your local hardware store (this may surprise you, but hardware stores, such as Ace, often have canning sections and are good sources for jars and other equipment).

Flavored salts can be used in fermentation, assuming they are free of chemical additives. If they are cut with a significant amount of herbs or spices, you should increase the salt quantity in your recipe to account for the lower sodium chloride content. That is the main downside to flavored salt: you really have no idea how much of the salt, by weight, is cut with the flavoring agents, which makes it more difficult to get really accurate salt percentages. While you can use these salts to add flavor to your ferments, we encourage you to use an unflavored salt, which is more predictable, and simply add herbs and spices to your ferments to achieve the desired flavor.

Smoked salt is exactly that: salt that has been smoked. These salts can be used for fermentation and will add a touch of smoky flavor to the finished ferment. The smokiness will likely be dulled by the fermentation process, but some smoky flavor will come through in the end result.

Kosher salt is another highly refined salt. It is usually coarse grained and sometimes contains additives such as anticaking agents. You can use this salt for fermenting, but be sure to check the label to make sure it is additive-free.

Real Salt is a brand of mineral salt mined from an ancient salt deposit near Redmond, Utah. This salt deposit was left behind from an ancient sea that covered North America millions of years ago. Real Salt has a slight pink hue, similar to Himalayan pink salt, and contains over sixty trace minerals, making it an excellent domestic salt for all your ferments.

These are just a handful of the salts available worldwide. There are many, many more, each with their own production process, and each containing different minerals. Ultimately, the choice of which to use is up to you. Just make sure to check the label to ensure that there are no additives—salt should be the only ingredient listed.

WATER

Water is an important element of fermentation. The water you use in a ferment will have an impact on the microbes and, ultimately, the finished flavor of that ferment.

For brined ferments, sour tonics, kombucha, water kefir, and any alcohol ferment to which water is added, you can use distilled water, reverse osmosis purified water, spring water, well water, or filtered tap water. The main thing to remember is never to use *unfiltered* city tap water for any of the aforementioned ferments. Municipal tap water is chlorinated, which will have an adverse effect on the organisms needed for fermentation. Chlorinated water can harm the cultures in SCOBY ferments like kombucha and water kefir so much as to render them inviable. That being said, filtered tap water is fine, or you can let unfiltered tap water sit out open to the air for twenty-four to forty-eight hours, which will allow the chlorine to evaporate. For lightly rinsing produce, any type of water is fine.

Highly purified water, such as distilled, reverse osmosis, or home-filtered water, is preferable to unfiltered tap water, but these waters lack minerals that assist in the fermentation process. For most brined fruits and vegetables, this is not much of an issue because the produce itself adds minerals to the ferment. For kombucha and water kefir, however, using highly filtered water with no minerals can have a detrimental effect on the fermentation organisms over time, resulting in sluggish growth of the SCOBY. This lack of minerals can be overcome by the addition of dried fruit, mineral drops, or baking soda, or the use of coconut water or coconut sugar (see variations, page 316), which contain significant minerals.

PRODUCE: CALCULATING WASTE AND PURCHASE QUANTITIES

For all the ferments in this book, we have listed the exact quantity of produce you will need to fill the specified jar. Our recipes are designed to fill jars as much as possible while still maintaining adequate headspace (2 inches). Proper fill rates are important for limiting oxygen in the jar because too much oxygen can lead to contamination. But the quantities we have specified are the net amounts going *into* the jar, *not* the amounts you need to purchase. When you prep fruits and vegetables—core a cabbage, peel ginger, etc.—there will almost always be waste as a result. The waste percentages are highly variable, so to make sure you're buying or otherwise procuring the right gross quantity of produce, you need to know the approximate waste percentages of each fruit or vegetable. There are numerous online resources for gathering waste and yield percentages on produce. Just remember that it is always optimal to buy more produce than needed to avoid coming up short. With most produce, the waste is insignificant enough that you just need to buy a little extra, but with items like cabbage, which has a higher waste yield, it is more important to understand the concept of waste and yield in order to yield the proper quantities.

For example, the Basic Kraut recipe (page 92) calls for 1,960 grams of cabbage. (We use grams and milliliters instead of kilograms and liters in order to make the math easier.) Cabbage waste is typically around 15 percent, though less-dense, leafy heads can be as high as 20 percent. To accommodate for this waste and to buy the right amount in order to fill the jar for the basic kraut recipe, the equation would look like this:

Net cabbage desired = 1,960 grams ÷ 454 [grams per pound]
    = 4.3 pounds
Gross cabbage to purchase = 4.3 pounds x 1.2 [20% waste]
    = 5.16 pounds

Once you have the gross purchase quantity, round up to make sure you don't end up short—in the example above, round 5.16 pounds up to 5.5 pounds to ensure you'll have the desired net quantity. We've given this example because while all our recipes are in metric, almost all grocery store scales are measured in pounds, so you'll need to convert the grams into pounds for shopping purposes.

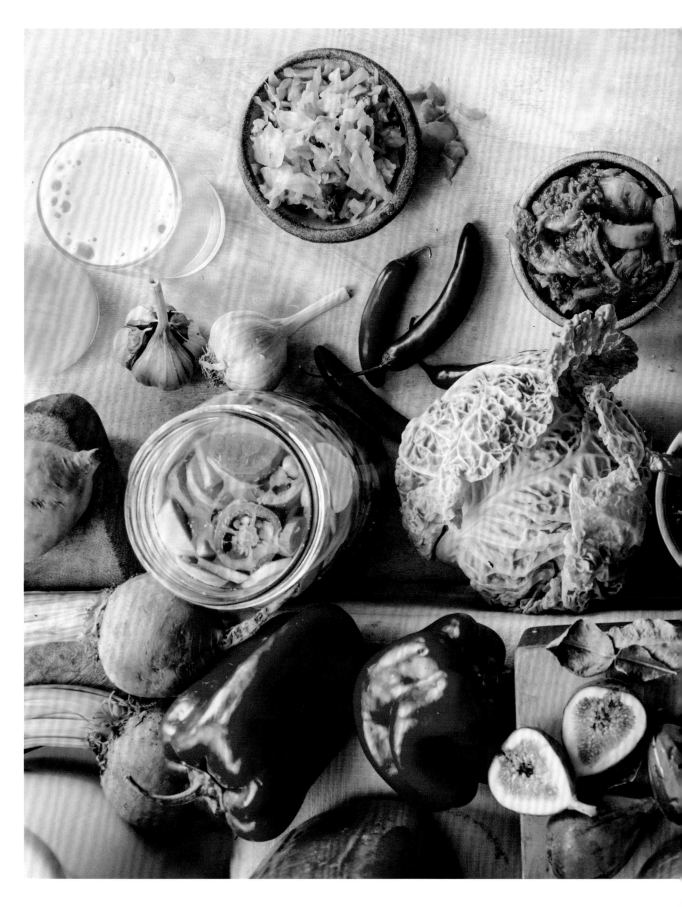

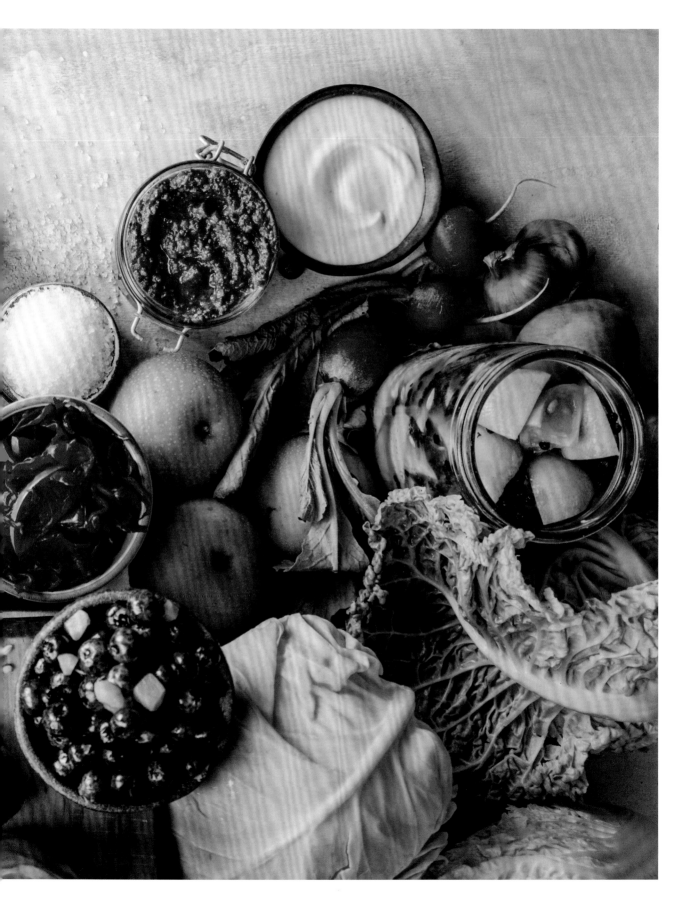

STARTER CULTURES, WILD FERMENTS, AND NATIVE MICROBES

On the backs of microbes, humanity's most intriguing and flavorful foods are forged. Whether relying on yeast, mold, or bacteria, the conclusion is the same: without the powerful transformative power of these tiny little beings, human civilization would be far less evolved and nourished. These magical microbes, our cohorts in fermentation, have enabled us to pre-serve the bounty of the forests and the fields for millennia. As science throws light on these shadowy little figures and our understanding of the Microcosmos expands, we are gaining more and more insight into how these microbes play a vital role in everything from forest ecosystems to our own human ecosystem. Whether you're using a starter culture or relying on native microbes (as with wild ferments), your microbial partners in fermen-tation are a complex and indelible part of fermentation. The term *starter culture* is used to describe a catalyst of fermentation, any substance that contributes a significant source of bacterial, yeast, or mold cultures to a fer-ment, which will initiate and perpetuate the fermentation process. There are a number of starter cultures that you can employ to get your ferments on the path to transformation, or you can simply ferment them wildly.

Lactic Acid Bacteria

Lactic acid bacteria (LAB) starter cultures come in many forms: kraut brine, pickle brines, rejuvelac, whey, and cabbage juice all are high in LAB and can be used to culture fruits, vegetables, and more. You can also buy powdered LAB starter cultures, but it is really unnecessary to do so. All vegetables and fruits have LAB on their skins or leaves in varying degrees. Most vegetables don't need a starter culture because the vegetables them-selves are covered in LAB, which, given the right environment, will initiate spontaneous fermentation (also called wild fermentation). To lacto-ferment fruit, however, starter cultures are essential for giving the LAB an advan-tage over the wild yeasts that seek to transform the fruit's sugar into alcohol instead of lactic acid. Using any of the starter cultures listed above and a little bit of salt, you can lacto-ferment all kinds of fruits, creating delicious and unique flavor profiles and giving you another tool to preserve the bounty of the seasons.

For many of the recipes in this book, we have used kraut brine as a starter culture. The main reason we have done this is to show you both the wild and cultured methods, but also to illustrate that you can get away with using less salt if you employ some type of starter culture, as with our brined ferments. It is important to use a wild ferment, such as kraut, as your starter culture, because you can have issues if you continue to culture batches with other cultured batches. For example, if you used a kraut brine to start your next batch of kraut, and you continued to use each subsequent batch as the starter for the next, over time the bacteria can develop a sickness called bacteriophage, ultimately resulting in the loss of bacterial diversity and in sickly, failed batches of kraut. Kraut does not need a starter culture because cabbage is naturally covered in diverse populations of lactic acid bacteria and does not generally benefit from the use of a starter culture.

We try to use wild fermentation whenever we can. Using the indigenous microflora on your produce will, in essence, create unique place-based ferments that are full of bacterial biodiversity. This biodiversity not only creates a healthier and more productive ecosystem in your crock or jar, but also results in you, the consumer, digesting and reaping the benefits of all that biodiversity. We have used wild fermentation in many of the recipes, including all of the krauts, kimchi, and pepper mashes, to show you how simple and low-input fermentation can be. All you need are salt, vegetables, and time. It's truly that simple.

Yeast Starter Culture Varieties and Wild Methods

While the bacterial starter cultures are few, yeast starters are far more varied and diverse. When discussing the yeast used in any alcohol ferment, we are talking about the species *Saccharomyces cerevisiae*. Within that species, there are literally hundreds of different strains to choose from, so many that we can't even begin to scratch the surface here. You can buy powdered or liquid yeast at any brewing supply store or online quite cheaply (around $1 per packet of powdered yeast, a bit more for the liquid versions). Each yeast producer has extensive explanations of their yeast strains on their website, with information about how the strain performs in fermentation; the flavor and aroma it produces in the finished drink; and its flocculation rates, temperature requirements, and sugar and alcohol tolerances. These are the main points to note when choosing a yeast strain for your home ferments.

If you are confused about which strain to use, we encourage you to ask the experts at your local brewing supply shop, or do some research online, where you can find detailed information about each type of yeast. While it's not possible to go into all the available yeast strains, here are a few favorites.

Champagne yeast is great for most of my (Shane's) meads, and especially good for dry sparkling meads and sparkling hard ciders. There are many Champagne yeasts, but I typically use the Lalvin EC-1118, which blueberries are three fruits that come to mind that have visible blooms on their skins, and they are probably the three best fruits for culturing unfermented must with native or wild yeasts (though all fruits will have some wild yeast on their skins to varying degrees, so don't feel limited to these three). The best method for culturing your alcohol using these fruits is to prepare the must in an open-top fermenter (any vessel without a lid or seal can be used), add the fruit, and cover with a porous cloth such as cheesecloth. The action of the wild yeast should be visible after three to four days: you should see the ferment bubbling vigorously, which tells you the wild yeasts are active and that it is time to rack the must into a carboy, leaving the fruit behind. This is essentially the same process used for the primary fermentation in winemaking. Note that while yeast on the skins of fruit you buy from the grocery store will technically be wild yeast strains, they likely won't be local strains (unless, of course, they were grown locally).

Yeast Nutrients

Just like all living things, yeast needs nutrients to grow healthy, proliferate, and produce the desired outcome of alcohol production. For this reason adding a small amount of yeast nutrient can positively affect the outcome of your alcohol ferments. Some packets of yeast come with added nutrients in the powdered culture, while others do not. When purchasing the yeast for your alcohol production, check to see if the yeast you have chosen contains nutrients or not. If it does not, you can choose from a wide variety of yeast nutrients, available online or at brewing supply stores. You only need a very small amount of this stuff, as a little goes a long way, but it makes a big difference and results in a more rapid fermentation. I've been using the yeast nutrient BSG Superfood by CraftBrewing with much success, so this is the nutrient that's been called out in the recipes, but you can successfully use a number of different yeast nutrients.

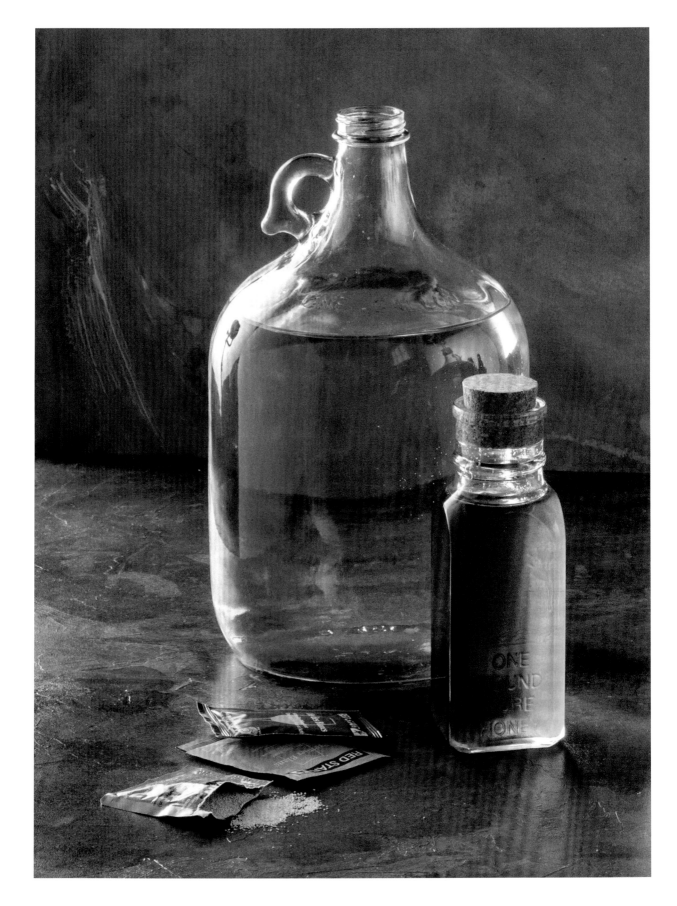

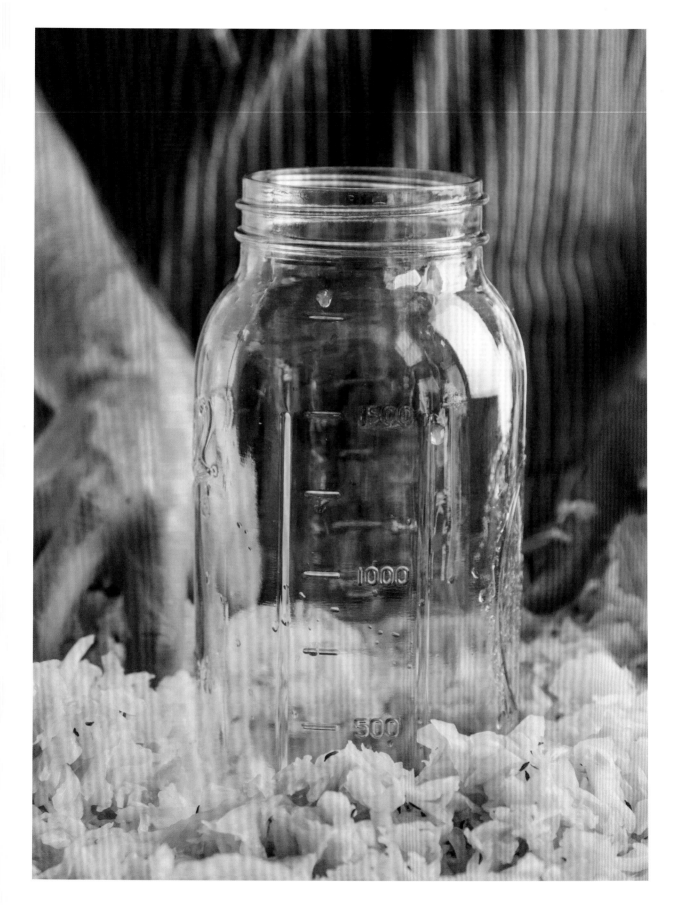

is always better and more accurate than volume, and metric weights and volumes allow the fermenter to be more precise. While humans have been fermenting for thousands of years without the use of scales, it was a craft that was handed down from generation to generation that supplied the knowledge enabling them to get the right amount of salt into their ferments, likely by taste. We highly advise the beginning fermenter to weigh out your ingredients every time, tasting the unfermented mixtures so that you know what it should taste like. Once you know the proper taste, you can eyeball the ingredients if you prefer. The salt level of most ferments should taste close to that of ocean water (ocean salinity varies but is typically 2.5 to 3.5%), almost too salty to the palate but not quite.

If you decide to experiment with fermenting vegetables other than those found in this book, here is a useful tip: For dry-salted vegetables, roughly 1,000 grams will fill a 1-liter jar (946 grams of vegetables will fill a 1-quart jar). For brining, a good rule to follow is 45% solids (fruits or vegetables) to 55% brine.

It may not seem so, but the difference between 2% salt and 3% salt can be huge, and the smaller the batch size, the more accurate your weighed measurements need to be. For instance, when you're making a large crock or barrel of kraut, being off by a few grams won't alter the percentage significantly or affect the outcome of the ferment, but being off by a few grams in a 1- or 2-liter batch can alter the salt percentage significantly. We think lack of accuracy with salt, along with inadequately sealed vessels, are the main reasons beginning home fermenters have higher rates of failed batches than the experienced fermenter will encounter.

Last, it should be noted here that many people use baker's percentages instead of true percentages when calculating salt and brine percentages for fermentation recipes. We use true percentages in all of our recipes to achieve the most accurate salt percentages, offering you the best chance at success with your home ferments. Using baker's percentages can be useful when you are in the kitchen and need to figure out some quick math on the fly, or you have an odd amount of produce and need to quickly figure out the salt quantity, but it is less accurate. For example, if you want to make 1 liter of kraut at 2% salt strength, using baker's percentages you would multiply 1,000 by 2% to figure out your salt quantity, which would yield a ratio of 1,000 grams cabbage to 20 grams salt. It seems logical, but in fact with this ratio you will have less than 2% salt in the finished kraut because the total grams is now 1,020 grams. The same equation using a true percentage would actually have a ratio of 980 grams cabbage to 20 grams salt, equaling 1,000 grams or 1 liter total. The difference is small, both methods can be used, but using true percentages is more accurate.

TIME AND TEMPERATURE

When it comes to fermentation, time and temperature are inseparable, and they cannot be explained separately because they are directly correlated. Whether we're talking about lactic acid, SCOBY, alcohol, or yogurt fermentation, the same basic principle applies: the warmer the temperature, the faster the ferment will progress, and vice versa. The fermentation time tables in each recipe in this book are meant to be used as guidelines and to provide insight into this time-temperature relationship, but they're not exact. There are many factors at play—like salt quantity (see "Kitchen Scale," page 55), the amount of sugars available for the microbes to digest, and the species and quantity of microbes present in your crock or carboy—so giving exact fermentation times is very difficult. Also, because the home fermenter will likely be unable to keep a steady temperature during both day and night, guesstimating the fermentation time is essentially impossible.

One of the nuanced aspects of fermentation that you will have to face is finding suitable environments to accommodate the different microbial temperature preferences for each style of ferment. Every home is different, and every homeowner has a different climate outside their home, which they are trying to counteract with heating and air conditioning. It's up to you to find the little microclimates in your home that will facilitate the proper temperature for your ferments. For example, if you keep your home at a steady 68°F, you'll likely be able to find a corner, far away from the central heating, that is cooler than the rest of your home. This would be an ideal place to ferment your lacto-ferments, such as kraut and kimchi.

Just as with gardening, where it can take years to fully understand all the microclimates on your property and the best place to grow each type of plant, understanding the microclimates in your home can take some time. It's worth investing in an electronic temperature gauge or thermometer that you can place in different parts of your home and keep an eye on to understand where the cold and warm pockets are. To give you an example, at the property where we homesteaded for many years, after much observation we were able to find a cold shed that stayed shaded in the summer, resulting in a nice, cool climate even when temperatures outside were soaring. This is where Shane did a lot of fermentation in the summer, but in the winter, it got far too cold for anything other than storing homemade hooch, kraut, and such. Conversely, the garage on the property was far too hot for fermentation in the summer, but stayed a steady cool (but not too cold) temperature during winter.

"Between fresh and rotten, there's a creative space where some of the most compelling flavors arise."

—SANDOR ELLIX KATZ

DIY Fermentoriums

A fermentorium is any space that is designated for fermentation, often but not always implementing a climate-controlled atmosphere to maintain proper fermentation temperature and humidity. You can make your own DIY fermentorium with a few basic tools and little effort.

For alcohol ferments, which typically do best at temperatures around 70°F, you can purchase **carboy heaters**, which are flexible and wrap around the carboy. These will typically raise the temperature enough to be able to ferment during the cold winter months.

Similarly, you can buy **seedling sprouting mats** at most garden supply stores or plant nurseries. These thin electric heat mats will raise the ambient temperature about 10°F above the temperature of the room, and we use them because they are cheap and effective. For kombucha, which can take very long to ferment in cold temperatures and benefits from a steady temperature between 70° and 80°F, the use of heating mats is a necessity if you're fermenting during cold winter months. We place fermenting kombucha in a cabinet with a heating mat, and successfully ferment kombucha year-round. You can also use these mats for any other ferment which needs a warmer climate. **Insulated coolers** can also easily be turned into DIY fermentoriums using a heating mat.

With a temperature gauge and a heating mat, you can turn any space into a DIY fermentorium, but if you want to devote a larger space to fermentation, you will need to purchase a larger heating unit. I (Shane) have many years of experience building fermentoriums, and have also built greenhouses and designed their heating/cooling systems. There is actually quite a bit of overlap between these two systems, as they both seek to maintain a constant temperature and climate within. The simplest way to turn a room in your house into a fermentorium is to buy a thermostat (available at hydroponic or home improvement stores) into which you can plug a heater and air conditioner, purchase a small heating and/or AC unit, depending on your climate needs, then simply plug in the heater and AC and set the temperature to your desired setting. This system, while costly, will ensure that temperature is maintained through cold and warm spells and will also keep the climate constant through day and night temperature swings.

But most people don't have an entire room to devote to fermentation, and if you do, you probably don't want to pay to heat and cool the entire space when your ferments only take up a portion of the room. To reduce the space, you can build a fermentation box out of plywood, make faux walls out of plastic or cardboard, or simply turn an old piece of furniture such as a cabinet or hutch into a fermentation space. Limiting the space you have to heat or cool will lower the cost of doing so and will also make it easier and faster to heat or cool the space.

All that being said, often all you need to do is find the right warm or cool space in your home to place your ferments, and forgo the cost and effort of building a fermentorium.

Troubleshooting: When Bad Things Happen to Good Ferments

Leaving food on your counter to ferment takes some getting used to. It goes against everything we've been taught about food safety. While our Pasteurian ways may lead us to be fearful of such practices, we can assure you that fermentation is a safe and reliable method of preservation that has been used for thousands of years. In properly fermented mediums, the metabolic action of the bacteria and yeast effectively preserves your ferment using either lactic acid or ethanol, rendering the medium nearly impossible for pathogenic organisms to colonize.

Armed with information and your senses of smell, taste, and sight, you can safely and effectively ferment countless types of foods and beverages. Proper sanitization, adequate salt concentrations, and making sure that your ferments are anaerobic and sufficiently submerged under the brine will contribute to the success of your home ferments. As the famous saying by Benjamin Franklin goes, "An ounce of prevention is worth a pound of cure," and this is very appropriate when talking about fermentation defects. But sometimes, despite your best efforts, things can go wrong. Here are some common maladies and how to handle them.

Foam present on top of your ferments is not a defect and does not need to be removed. This is a normal part of the LAB fermentation process and is a result of the heterofermentative microbes producing gases. Let it be—the foaming will eventually subside.

White film on the surface is a common defect in fermented fruits and vegetables and is a result of contamination by yeasts, most often Kahm yeast. While this yeast will produce bready off flavors that you may find off-putting, rest assured that below that layer of white film often lies a delicious ferment. Use a clean sterilized spoon to scrape off the top layer, removing as much of the film as you can. The ferment is still totally safe to consume—you can decide whether you like the taste. We just don't like the flavors produced by this yeast, so we usually toss out the ferment if the bready flavor is still there after scraping, but many people can tolerate or even like it.

Mold is quite different from yeast and can produce toxins that are unhealthy for humans to consume. We've all seen mold growing on foods, and although there are many varieties of mold, you should be able to easily tell mold apart from other contaminating organisms, such as yeast. Mold usually just infects the upper reaches of a ferment. With kraut and other dry-salted vegetables, you can usually get away with scraping off a good portion of the top layer of the ferment; the vegetables below are often fine and tasty. If you find mold growing on the surface of liquid mediums, such as sour tonics or brined vegetables, you should throw out the ferment. Mold can send filaments called hyphae down into the ferment and create toxic substances that you shouldn't be eating. Some fermenters take a laissez-faire approach to mold, but we take it quite seriously and almost always toss a moldy batch on the compost heap. If you find mold growing on a kombucha mother, the verdict is the same: toss it and reevaluate your fermentation practices.

Pink kraut is a rare defect. It has typically been observed in kraut with an abnormally high salt content, above 2.5%. The pink hue can be attributed to the growth of pigmented yeast. Pink kraut, while safe to consume, will likely have off flavors—in Kathryn's early days of fermenting, she made a kraut that was tinged pink and tasted like fish. We recommend throwing out pink kraut or feeding it to the chickens.

If you find that your fermented **vegetables are slimy** or the **brine is viscous**, this is likely due to dextran, a naturally occurring polysaccharide (sugar). When the bacteria set out to ferment a medium, they must first break down the glucose into sucrose and fructose. During this process, dextran strands are produced, which create a slimy texture in the ferment. This often happens at higher fermentation temperatures. Don't fret—the dextran strands will eventually be broken down and the slimy texture will go away. Simply continue to ferment the mixture for another week or so, at which time the sliminess should be gone and a perfectly good ferment will endure.

Softening in kraut or fermented vegetables is a common defect. All vegetable ferments will lose their crunchy texture and go soft over time as a result of the breakdown of the pectic walls that create that texture to begin with. Watery vegetables, such as cucumbers (which also have softening enzymes present on their skins), have a tendency to go soft sooner.

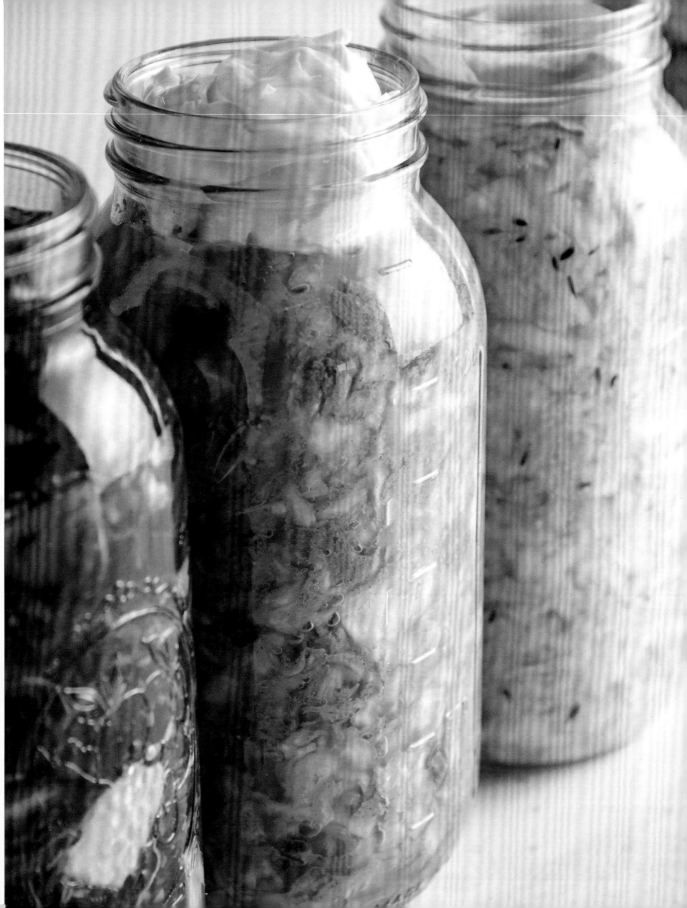

Kraut

There is nothing quite as tasty as freshly fermented kraut. Pleasingly tart and full of crunch, it bears little resemblance to its canned counterpart. My (Kathryn's) first batch in 2004 was made somewhat haphazardly, and I was pretty nervous as I watched it bubbling away on my counter. I found it hard to wrap my head around the fact that just two simple ingredients, cabbage and salt, could be transformed by "unseen forces" into a safe and delicious food. But transform they did indeed, and I was immediately hooked.

We often recommend that fermentation newbies start with kraut. It is almost impossible to screw up, and getting that first successful batch under your belt can provide the confidence needed to move on to more adventurous ferments. Follow our instructions and you'll soon be fermenting your own kraut with great success.

FERMENTER'S NOTES

Produce: Cabbage leaves are particularly high in populations of lactic acid bacteria (LAB) and as a result, kraut requires no starter culture. This is equally true of all cabbage, of which there are countless varieties, some even grown specifically for kraut making. The fresher the cabbage, the higher the LAB count, so look for dense heads with shiny leaves. Also, keep in mind when you're shopping that the waste percentage when processing cabbage is between 15 and 20%. This means you will need to purchase 15 to 20% more cabbage than is specified in the following recipes.

When selecting other vegetables, aromatics, and herbs for your kraut, make sure they are fresh and of high quality, as produce that has bruises or cuts could be harboring yeasts or mold and should be avoided. Once you realize how easy it is to make delicious kraut at home, you may want to expand your kraut making to other recipes beyond what's included in this book. If you should choose to venture out with your own kraut recipes, we recommend that the total weight of vegetables, herbs, and spices other than cabbage not exceed 25% of the total recipe weight. Since cabbage is such a great catalyst for fermentation, keeping the cabbage quantity at 75% or more of the total recipe will ensure a higher success rate with a variable array of delicious krauts. Farmers' markets can be a great source of inspiration for cabbage and other kraut ingredients, plus you know you're getting the freshest produce possible.

Prepping the cabbage: Most often, cabbage does not need to be rinsed unless it is especially dirty. Remove the outer leaves until clean, shiny leaves are revealed. Set aside two of the outer leaves for later use, to be folded and added to the mouth of the canning jar. (The folded-up cabbage leaf serves two purposes—it protects the shredded cabbage below from oxygen in case of a breach in the airlock or lid, and it applies downward pressure on the mixture so the solids stay submerged below the brine.) Cut the head in half (or into quarters, if it's large) and make a V-shaped cut around the core on each half. Use the tip of the knife to pry out the core. Place the halved heads cut-side down on your cutting surface. Slice the cabbage into ⅛- to ¼-inch-thick shreds. (The size of the shred is, to some degree, a matter of preference. We prefer a finer shred but there are home fermenters who favor a thicker shred.) As soon as your cabbage is cut, the sugars within are exposed to the atmosphere and unwanted microbes. Work diligently to limit the time the cut cabbage sits out, and get it salted, mixed, and in your jar as soon as possible to avoid contamination from airborne microbes.

Salt: The accepted range of salt for kraut is 1.5 to 2.5% by weight. We've experimented with the full range of salt percentages and have found that 2% consistently yields the best flavor and texture. In warmer temperatures, which can favor the growth of yeast, the salt can be increased to as high as 2.5% to slow down the fermentation process and favor LAB. Conversely, if fermenting in cold temperatures, which can slow fermentation time, the salt can be decreased to as low as 1.5% in order to speed up fermentation.

Brine: The water content of a cabbage can vary due to season, growing practices, and variety. If your cabbage does not initially produce enough liquid to fully submerge the vegetable, you can make extra brine to top it off—in most cases, 100 grams of brine should be enough. Simply dissolve 2 grams salt in 98 milliliters filtered water and top the kraut off with the brine, leaving 2 inches of headspace in the jar. This brine can also be used if you lose some of the brine through the airlock or lid during the fermentation process.

If this happens, open the jar, add the replacement brine, again leaving 2 inches of headspace, and reseal (leave the jar open only as long as it takes to add the brine, to avoid introducing unwanted yeasts and molds). During the first five to seven days, gas (CO_2) is produced, which can cause the brine to be expelled through the airlock, potentially dropping the brine level below the vegetables. If you add replacement brine too soon, it will just be expelled by the gases, too, so wait until the end of this first phase before adding more brine. The exposed vegetables are protected by a layer of CO_2 during this phase and generally will not deteriorate. You'll know this phase is complete when the airlock stops bubbling.

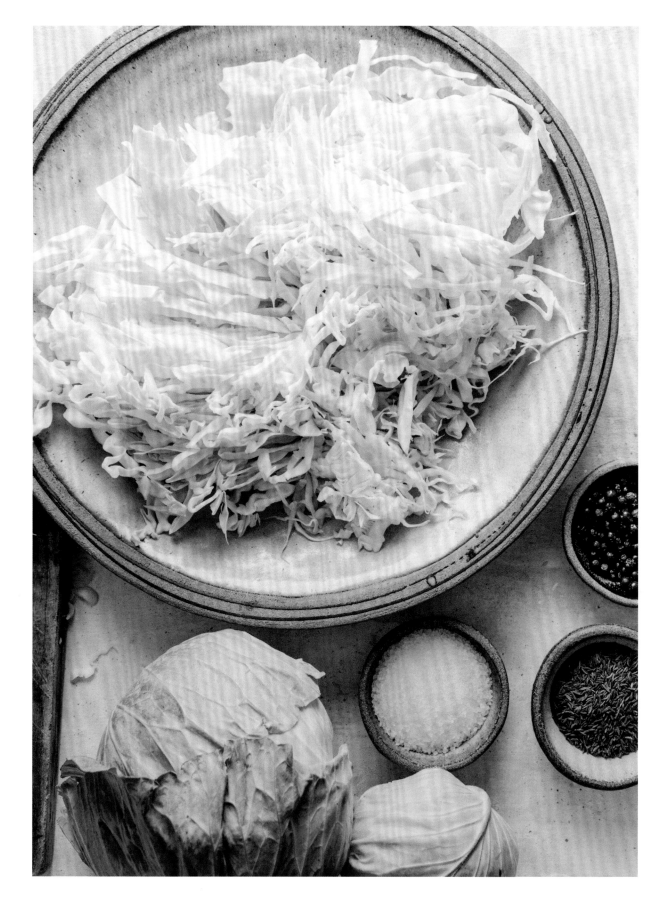

BASIC KRAUT

1,960 grams shredded green, white, or red cabbage (⅛- to ¼-inch-thick shreds)

40 grams coarse unrefined sea salt

1 tablespoon caraway seeds or juniper berries (optional)

2 whole cabbage leaves

EQUIPMENT

Kitchen scale

½-gallon or 2-liter wide-mouth glass jar

Canning funnel (optional)

Kraut tamper (optional)

Fermentation lid

Fermentation Temperature & Time

Above 68°F
Ferment 2 weeks or less

65° to 68°F
Ferment 2 to 3 weeks

Ideal: 64°F
Ferment 3 weeks

60° to 63°F
Ferment 3 to 4 weeks

Below 60°F
Ferment 4 weeks or more

Caraway and juniper berries are both classic additions to traditional Bavarian-style kraut. We love both, but have a slight preference for caraway because of its carminative (gas-preventing) properties. With that said, we typically make our basic kraut "naked" because we use it so often to culture other foods and prefer to have a more blank flavor slate.

1. Wash and sanitize all your fermentation equipment, including a large bowl, knife, and cutting board, and set aside to air-dry.

2. Put the shredded cabbage in the large bowl and sprinkle the salt over the shredded cabbage, along with the caraway seeds or juniper berries. Using your hands, vigorously massage, squeeze, and mix the salt into the cabbage until the cabbage begins to release liquid, about 5 minutes. The cabbage will transform in color and texture, becoming more translucent and pliable as you go. When you can grab a handful of the shredded cabbage and squeeze the liquid out of it easily, it's ready to go.

3. Transfer the cabbage to the jar along with the natural brine at the bottom of the bowl (a canning funnel is useful here and helps to minimize spillage). As you add the cabbage, tamp it down with your fist or a kraut tamper to submerge the solids under the brine and force out any air pockets. Continue until the jar is almost full, leaving 2 inches of headspace.

4. Take one of the two whole cabbage leaves, give it a quick rinse, and fold it up so it fits into the mouth of the jar.

It should cover all the cabbage below and very slightly protrude from the top of the jar. Depending on the size and density of the leaves, you may need to fold and add the second cabbage leaf if the kraut is not submerged under the brine when the lid is sealed.

5. Seal the jar with the fermentation lid. You should feel some resistance from the cabbage leaf, but not so much that tightening the lid is overly difficult. Place the sealed jar on a plate or in a bowl to catch any liquid displaced through the airlock during fermentation.

6. Ferment the kraut in a cool place away from direct sunlight (3 weeks at 64°F is ideal—see the chart at left). Taste the kraut after 2 weeks to determine if the flavor and sourness are to your liking. If it's not sour enough, reseal the jar and let it ferment for another week, then taste again. When the kraut is sour to your liking, replace the fermentation lid with a regular lid, seal, and store in the refrigerator for up to 10 months.

USING BASIC KRAUT AS A STARTER

Throughout this book, we have used this Basic Kraut recipe as the starter culture for fermenting other foods and drinks. This is because cabbage is a great catalyst for wild fermenting and capturing wild LAB—cabbage is easy to ferment, has a relatively neutral flavor that doesn't overpower the ferments its added to, and usually has a sufficient amount of inherent liquid that is transformed into a natural brine. We like to make batches of Basic Kraut just for the purpose of culturing our other ferments. When doing so, we prepare the kraut as stated in the recipe; however, we only allow it to ferment for 3 to 5 days, then move the jar into the refrigerator to slow down the fermentation process. This ultrashort fermentation time creates an underfermented kraut that is still high in populations of heterofermentative LAB. Moving the kraut to refrigeration slows the progress of the LAB down, but also favors the heterofermenters. This makes for a more optimal and diverse starter culture than a fully fermented batch of kraut, which contains mostly homofermentative LAB, namely *Lactobacillus*, producing a less nuanced and diverse fermented product. That being said, you can still use a fully fermented batch of kraut as your starter culture with much success, as it will still contain billions of LAB. In some of our recipes we call specifically for the natural brine from the Basic Kraut. If your kraut isn't very juicy, the best way to extract natural brine is to blend the kraut up into a slurry, and extract the natural brine through a sieve.

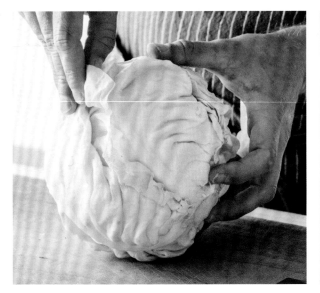 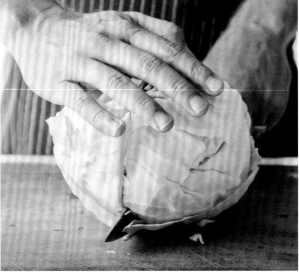

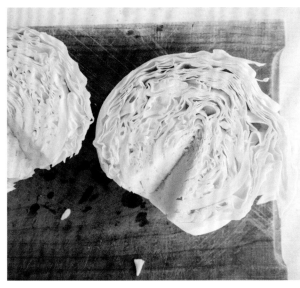 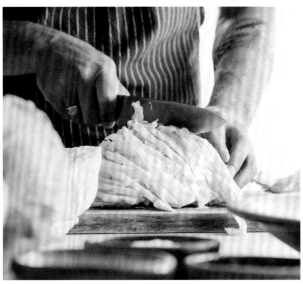

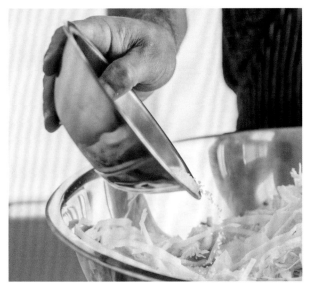 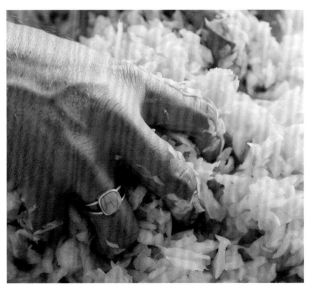

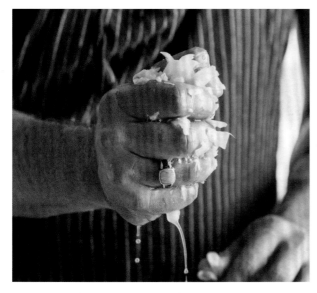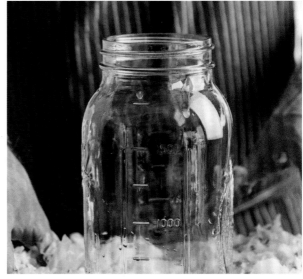

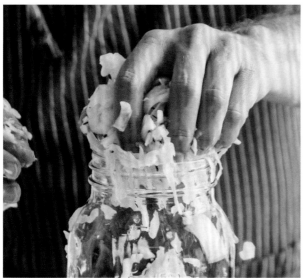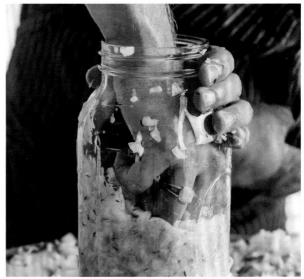

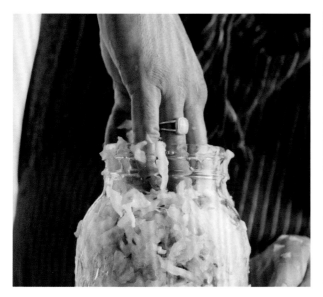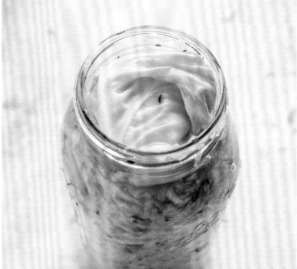

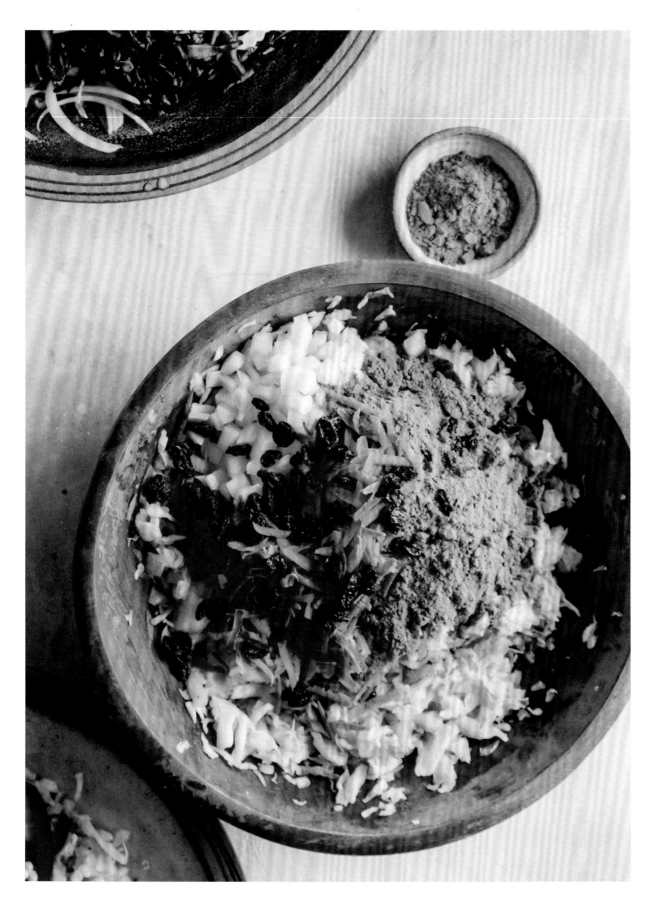

CURRIED KRAUT
with Raisins

MAKES ½ GALLON

1,620 grams shredded green cabbage (⅛- to ¼-inch-thick shreds)

40 grams coarse unrefined sea salt

150 grams shredded carrots

100 grams chopped white or yellow onion

50 grams raisins

40 grams curry powder

2 whole cabbage leaves

EQUIPMENT

Kitchen scale

½-gallon or 2-liter wide-mouth glass jar

Canning funnel (optional)

Kraut tamper (optional)

Fermentation lid

Because we adore Indian food, we've made several types of curried krauts through the years. Our favorite curry spice blend is muchi, because it is not quite as cumin-forward as some blends; it can be found online and in the bulk section of many natural food stores. You can, of course, use any curry blend you like. The bacteria gobble up most of the sugars in the raisins, so don't expect them to be sweet—instead, they are sour little balls of joy that pop in your mouth and may become your favorite part of this kraut.

We've kept the ingredients in this recipe simple so you can easily add any number of fresh vegetables—just reduce the amount of cabbage by the amount of vegetables you're adding (and remember not to add more than 25% by weight). Some of our favorites include cauliflower, broccoli, and zucchini. Keep in mind that broccoli and cauliflower are bulky, so you may need to chop them into small florets in order to get all the vegetables into your jar.

This kraut is absolutely spectacular chopped and added to a curried chicken salad.

1. Wash and sanitize all your fermentation equipment, including a large bowl, knife, and cutting board, and set aside to air-dry.

2. Put the shredded cabbage in the large bowl and sprinkle the salt over the shredded cabbage. Using your hands, vigorously massage, squeeze, and mix the salt into the cabbage until the cabbage begins to release liquid, about 5 minutes. The cabbage will transform in color and texture, becoming more translucent and pliable as you go. When you can grab a handful of the shredded cabbage and squeeze the liquid out of it easily, it's ready to go. Add the carrots, onion, raisins, and curry powder to the bowl with the cabbage and mix to combine.

3. Transfer the mixture to the jar along with the natural brine at the bottom of the bowl (a canning funnel is useful here and helps to minimize spillage). As you add the mixture, tamp it down with your fist or a kraut tamper to submerge the solids under the brine and force out any air pockets. Continue until the jar is almost full, leaving 2 inches of headspace.

·CONTINUED ›

density of the leaves, you may need to fold and add the second cabbage leaf if the kraut is not submerged under the brine when the lid is sealed.

5. Seal the jar with the fermentation lid. You should feel some resistance from the cabbage leaf, but not so much that tightening the lid is overly difficult. Place the sealed jar on a plate or in a bowl to catch any liquid displaced through the airlock during fermentation.

6. Ferment the kraut in a cool place away from direct sunlight (3 weeks at 64°F is ideal—see the chart on page 92). Taste the kraut after 2 weeks to determine if the flavor and sourness are to your liking. If it's not sour enough, reseal the jar and let it ferment for another week, then taste again. When the kraut is sour to your liking, replace the fermentation lid with a regular lid, seal, and store in the refrigerator for up to 10 months.

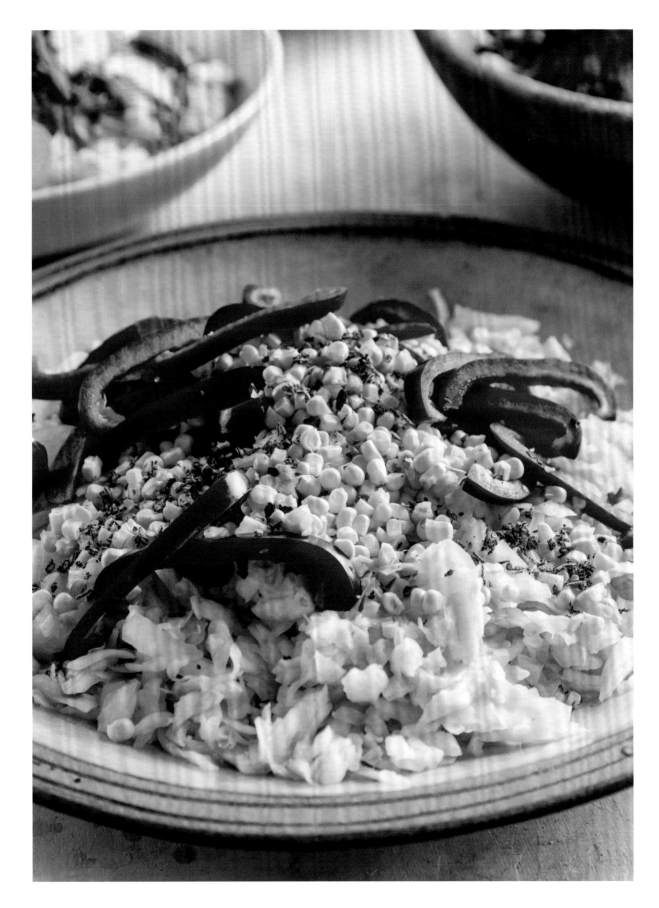

PAD THAI KRAUT

MAKES ½ GALLON

1,500 grams shredded green cabbage (⅛- to ¼-inch-thick shreds)

40 grams coarse unrefined sea salt

20 grams tamarind paste

20 grams fish sauce

Filtered water (as needed)

100 grams shredded carrots

100 grams thinly sliced radishes

100 grams chopped green onions (2-inch pieces)

60 grams bean sprouts

2 whole cabbage leaves

60 grams coarsely chopped roasted and salted peanuts for serving

EQUIPMENT

Kitchen scale

½-gallon or 2-liter wide-mouth glass jar

Canning funnel (optional)

Kraut tamper (optional)

Fermentation lid

In 2005, I attended the Blue Elephant Cooking School in Bangkok, where, in addition to learning how to make many traditional dishes, I discovered how to make the classic Thai noodle dish pad thai. A couple of years later, when I found myself topping a bowl of kraut with the pad thai vegetables and the sauce, skipping the noodles altogether, I had an aha moment: Why not add all the vegetables into the ferment? I did, and it worked beautifully, although Shane and I discovered when we developed this recipe that we preferred a slightly shorter fermenting time (14 days) to preserve the tamarind flavor.

Avoid fish sauces with additives—Red Boat fish sauce is generally considered the best and is readily available at most grocery stores. Tamarind paste is available at most grocery stores with an international or ethnic foods section. If you can't find it in the Asian section, check the Mexican foods section, as it's a common ingredient in Mexican cooking, too.

For a fun and satisfying side dish, toss this kraut with cooked fat rice noodles, top it with peanuts, and serve it with a wedge of lime for squeezing over the top. —Kathryn

1. Wash and sanitize all your fermentation equipment, including a large bowl, knife, and cutting board, and set aside to air-dry.

2. Put the shredded cabbage in the large bowl and sprinkle the salt over the shredded cabbage. Using your hands, vigorously massage, squeeze, and mix the salt into the cabbage until the cabbage begins to release liquid, about 5 minutes. The cabbage will transform in color and texture, becoming more translucent and pliable as you go. When you can grab a handful of the shredded cabbage and squeeze the liquid out of it easily, it's ready to go.

3. In a medium bowl, use a fork to mix the tamarind paste and fish sauce together. Add a few drops of filtered water, if needed, to loosen up the tamarind paste. Add the carrots, radishes, green onions, and bean sprouts and toss to coat with the tamarind mixture. Add the vegetables to the bowl with the cabbage and mix to combine.

4. Transfer the mixture to the jar along with the natural brine at the bottom of the bowl (a canning funnel is useful here and helps to minimize spillage). As you add the mixture, tamp it down with your fist or a kraut tamper to submerge the solids under the brine and

1,500 milliliters water

360 milliliters fresh lemon juice (from 7 to 9 lemons)

100 milliliters natural brine from Basic Kraut (page 92)

80 to 100 grams honey or 4 to 6 packets stevia

JULIANNE'S LIVE-CULTURE LEMONADE

My sister created this recipe in order to get more live cultures into her son's diet, but we all fell in love with it because it tastes so darned great. The kraut liquid actually accentuates the citrus notes while adding body to the lemonade. I'm not a fan of sugary drinks because they make me feel light-headed and giddy, but this lemonade has the opposite effect on me—it's really grounding. And because of the salt and the potassium in the kraut brine, it's also incredibly hydrating and nourishing in hot weather.

—Kathryn

To the water, add the lemon juice and the kraut brine. Stir until well combined. Add honey or stevia to taste. Serve over ice.

---

force out any air pockets. Continue until the jar is almost full, leaving 2 inches of headspace.

5. Take one of the two whole cabbage leaves, give it a quick rinse, and fold it up so it fits into the mouth of the jar. It should cover all the cabbage below and very slightly protrude from the top of the jar. Depending on the size and density of the leaves, you may need to fold and add the second cabbage leaf if the kraut is not submerged under the brine when the lid is sealed.

6. Seal the jar with the fermentation lid. You should feel some resistance from the cabbage leaf, but not so much that tightening the lid is overly difficult. Place the sealed jar on a plate or in a bowl to catch any liquid displaced through the airlock during fermentation.

7. Ferment the kraut in a cool place away from direct sunlight (3 weeks at 64°F is ideal—see the chart on page 92). Taste the kraut after 2 weeks to determine if the flavor and sourness are to your liking. If it's not sour enough, reseal the jar and let it ferment for another week, then taste again. When the kraut is sour to your liking, replace the fermentation lid with a regular lid, seal, and store in the refrigerator for up to 10 months. Garnish individual servings with chopped peanuts.

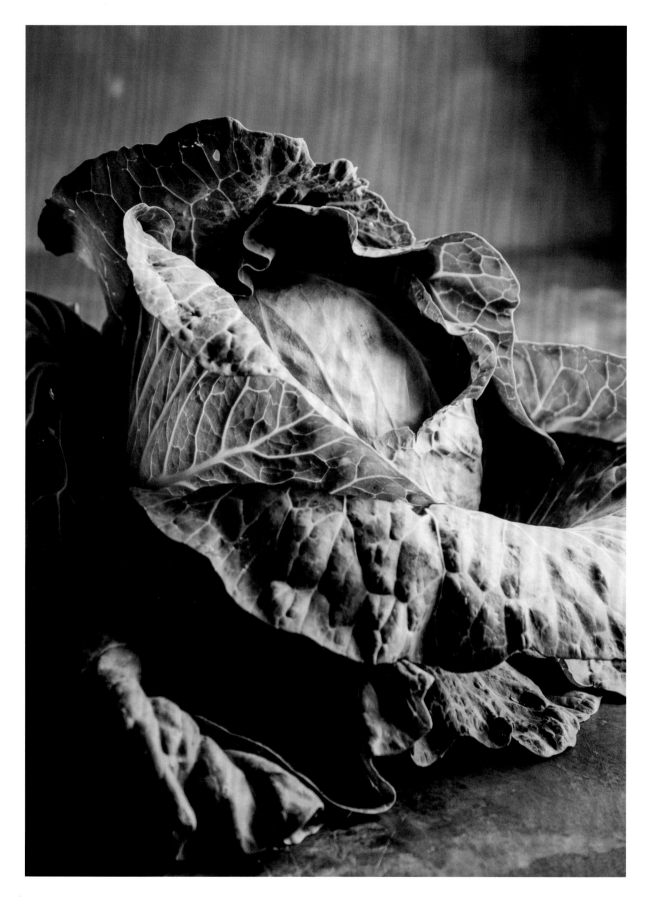

SURF-AND-TURF KRAUT

MAKES ½ GALLON

1,710 grams shredded green cabbage (⅛- to ¼-inch-thick shreds)

40 grams coarse unrefined sea salt

100 grams shredded carrots

100 grams chopped green onions (1- to 2-inch pieces)

30 grams mixed dried mushrooms (see headnote)

20 grams dried arame or wakame seaweed

2 whole cabbage leaves

EQUIPMENT

Kitchen scale

½-gallon or 2-liter wide-mouth glass jar

Canning funnel (optional)

Kraut tamper (optional)

Fermentation lid

You can use any type of dried mushroom successfully in this recipe. However, we discovered quite by (happy) accident that the combination of dried oyster, black trumpet, portobello, and porcini mushrooms along with dried arame seaweed come together to create a kraut that tastes like A.1. steak sauce. Strange but scrumptiously true!

1. Wash and sanitize all your fermentation equipment, including a large bowl, knife, and cutting board, and set aside to air-dry.

2. Put the shredded cabbage in the large bowl and sprinkle the salt over the shredded cabbage. Using your hands, vigorously massage, squeeze, and mix the salt into the cabbage until the cabbage begins to release liquid, about 5 minutes. The cabbage will transform in color and texture, becoming more translucent and pliable as you go. When you can grab a handful of the shredded cabbage and squeeze the liquid out of it easily, it's ready to go. Add the carrots, green onions, mushrooms, and seaweed to the bowl with the cabbage and mix to combine.

3. Transfer the mixture to the jar along with the natural brine at the bottom of the bowl (a canning funnel is useful here and helps to minimize spillage). As you add the mixture, tamp it down with your fist or a kraut tamper to submerge the solids under the brine and force out any air pockets. Continue until the jar is almost full, leaving 2 inches of headspace.

4. Take one of the two whole cabbage leaves, give it a quick rinse, and fold it up so it fits into the mouth of the jar. It should cover all the cabbage below and very slightly protrude from the top of the jar. Depending on the size and density of the leaves, you may need to fold and add the second cabbage leaf if the kraut is not submerged under the brine when the lid is sealed.

5. Seal the jar with the fermentation lid. You should feel some resistance from the cabbage leaf, but not so much that tightening the lid is overly difficult. Place the sealed jar in a bowl to catch any liquid displaced through the airlock during fermentation.

6. Ferment the kraut in a cool place away from direct sunlight (3 weeks at 64°F is ideal—see the chart on page 92). Taste the kraut after 2 weeks. If it's not sour enough, reseal the jar and let it ferment for another week, then taste again. When the kraut is sour to your liking, replace the fermentation lid with a regular lid, seal, and store in the refrigerator for up to 10 months.

5. Seal the jar with the fermentation lid. You should feel some resistance from the cabbage leaf, but not so much that tightening the lid is overly difficult. Place the sealed jar on a plate or in a bowl to catch any liquid displaced through the airlock during fermentation.

6. Ferment the kraut in a cool place away from direct sunlight (3 weeks at 64°F is ideal—see the chart on page 92). Taste the kraut after 2 weeks to determine if the flavor and sourness are to your liking. If it's not sour enough, reseal the jar and let it ferment for another week, then taste again. When the kraut is sour to your liking, replace the fermentation lid with a regular lid, seal, and store in the refrigerator for up to 10 months.

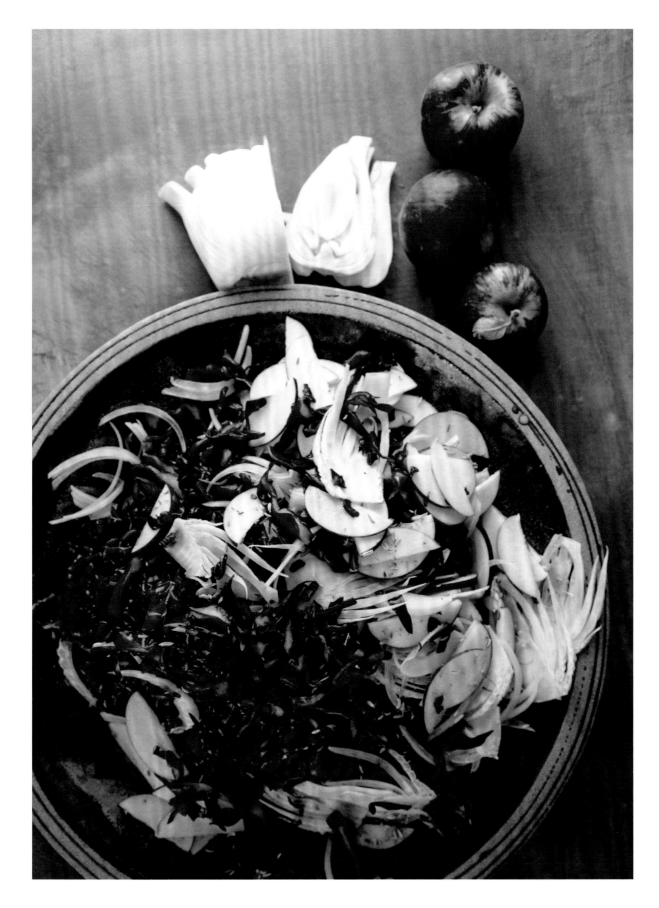

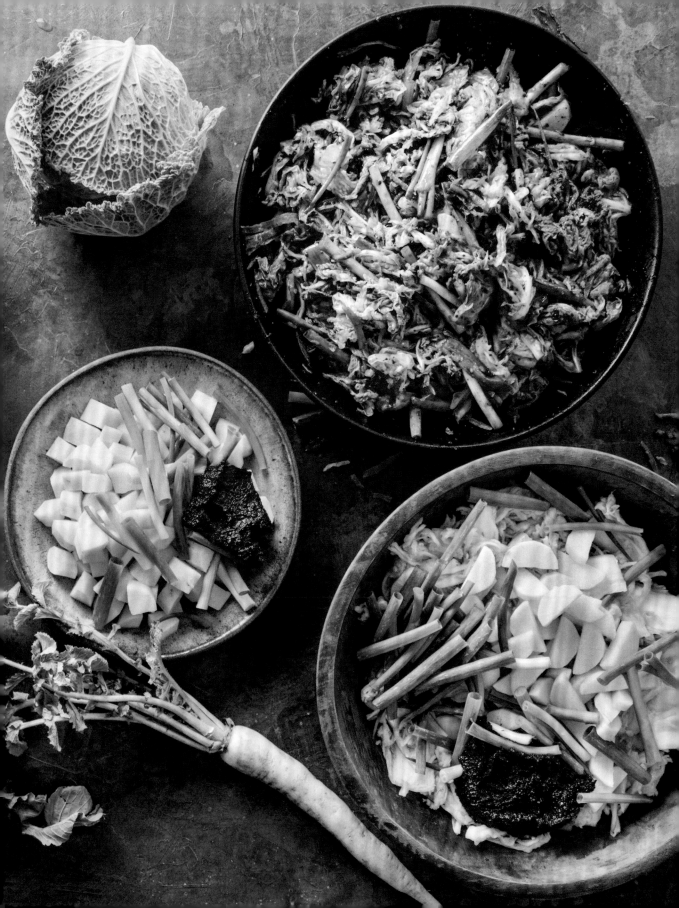

Kimchi

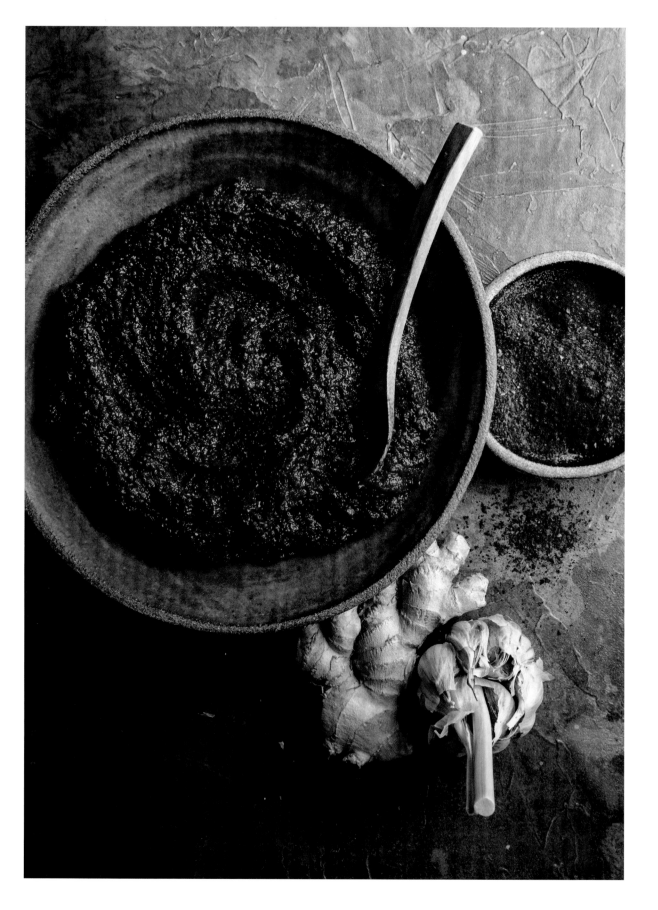

Kimchi, Korea's most iconic and culturally representative food, is likely the most diverse and widely varying group of ferments on the planet. The word *kimchi* is used to describe literally hundreds of different types of fermented products, everything from fruits, vegetables, and nuts to some varieties that contain raw fish, meat, and bone broth. There are around two hundred different varieties of kimchi nationally recognized in Korea. Within these, there are regional variations, and within those regional variations are seasonal and familial variations, as each family has their own recipes and techniques, passed down through generations. And even within these seasonal, regional, and familial variations, there are innumerable styles and subvariations—we are in awe of how diverse this ferment really is. *Baechu-kimchi*, a spicy cabbage ferment, is by far the most common style in both Korea and the US, and is the variety most often generically referred to as "kimchi." But to sum up the whole diverse range of this category of ferments by this one variety would be misguided.

For example, in the southern part of the Korean peninsula, with its close proximity to the sea and mild climate, seafood is often a component of kimchi and is typically quite spicy. In the northern part of the Korean peninsula, with its harsher and colder climate, and more limited access to fresh seafood, bone broth is often added to kimchi, and the kimchi is typically less spicy than it is in the south. Spring and summer kimchis are often eaten just barely fermented or served unfermented as a fresh salad. The vegetables are often elaborately cut and stuffed with salt and seasoning paste, resulting in beautiful and visually pleasing ferments like the summer cucumber kimchi called *oi-sobagi*. (While we appreciate the art of these beautifully crafted ferments, we've opted for more standard cuts for the vegetables in our recipes.) Fall kimchis are typically fermented over a much longer period, with more salt, which assists in the preservation of a longer ferment.

well in the fridge. It's also a delicious ingredient to cook with—we always have a jar of paste in the fridge to use for flavoring soups, stews, or any other recipe to which we want to add a touch of spice and umami.

Traditionally, kimchi paste is made by cooking sweet rice flour with water to make a gruel, which both thickens the paste and acts as an additional food source for the microbes in the ferment. Sugar is also added and assists in getting that effervescence into the finished kimchi, as well as feeding the microbes. Fish sauce and salted shrimp in the paste add flavor and umami to the finished kimchi. For our vegan, grain-free California-style paste, we opted to eliminate the rice gruel and to use dates instead of sugar as an additional food source for the microbes. We have used seaweed in place of the fish sauce and shrimp to give the paste that element of the ocean, and included dried mushrooms; both contribute their umami goodness to the final product.

If you want to get inspired to make kimchi, a trip to your local Korean market may be just the way to find that inspiration. Korean food culture is beautiful, and we highly encourage you to stoke this curiosity by paying your local Korean market a visit.

FERMENTER'S NOTES

Produce: Traditionally, napa or Chinese cabbage is used to make kimchi. While Chinese cabbage is very similar to napa, it is not as widely available. Both are less dense than European cabbage cultivars, and due to their higher water content, they produce significantly more brine. They also tend to be a lot buggier than other varieties, so make sure the heads are clean before you start.

Prepping the cabbage: Remove any dirty or yellow leaves. Remove and set aside two clean leaves for later use. Trim the stem end, quarter the head (through the stem end), and chop the cabbage into 2-inch square pieces. Add the cabbage to the bowl on the scale as you go until you have 1,400 grams; reserve any remaining cabbage for another use. Add the daikon, green onions, and salt to the bowl with the cabbage.

Salt: The accepted range of salt for kimchi is 1.5 to 2.5% by weight. All our kimchi recipes contain 2% salt by weight, which we have found consistently yields superior flavor and crunch. In warmer temperatures, which favor the growth of yeast, the salt can be increased to as high as 2.5% to slow down the fermentation process and favor lactic acid bacteria (LAB). Conversely, if fermenting in cold temperatures, which can slow fermentation time, the salt can be decreased to as low as 1.5% to speed up fermentation. Lower salt content and fermenting at lower temperatures both favor heterofermentative bacteria, resulting in a more flavorful kimchi.

Special ingredients: Before starting a kimchi recipe, familiarize yourself with these specialized ingredients. While most of these can be found online, Korean markets, which should be easy to find in most cities, are an excellent source for ingredients. They also sell traditional kimchis, which will give you an idea as to how yours should taste. When buying ingredients, it helps to know the Korean name of the ingredient in addition to its English translation, so there is no confusion and you end up with the right thing.

The main ingredient in kimchi paste, and the source of its heat, is **gochugaru**, or dried Korean chile pepper flakes. These spicy chile flakes are easily found in all Korean markets. They have a lovely flavor and mild to medium heat. *Gochugaru* is available in flake and powder form; opt for the flakes, if you can. They often stay fresher longer and ultimately add more flavor and spice. (We ordered *gochugaru* labeled "flakes" online, only to find when it arrived that it was, in fact, powdered, and it was not very flavorful.) As with all dried spices, freshness is key. Look for a vibrant red color; age and oxidation will start to turn the flakes or powder brownish or rusty red. If your *gochugaru* isn't very spicy, add some hot chile powder such as cayenne pepper to increase the heat of your paste. If using more cayenne, add to the paste in small increments of 10 grams or less as it can be easy to overdo it with this extremely spicy chile powder.

Sweet rice flour is widely available, both online and at many regular grocery stores. This flour is not the same as regular rice flour, so make sure it says "sweet" on the package. Regular rice flour is produced from long- to medium-grain rice, while sweet rice flour is produced from short-grain rice, which has a higher starch content and as a result is a better thickening agent. Blue Star Mochiko, made in California by Koda Farms, is a high-quality and widely available brand of sweet rice flour. We love that it is local, and used it for all our recipe development. There are other brands out there, including Bob's Red Mill and McCabe (the only organic brand we came across).

Salted shrimp, called *saeujeot* in Korean, are tiny little shrimp that are highly salted and very flavorful. They are usually found in the refrigerator section at Korean markets and contribute to the overall taste and umami of the paste and finished kimchi.

Fish sauce, called *jeotgal* in Korean, is a seasoning typically made from fermented anchovies. According to Lauryn Chun, author of *The Kimchi*

Cookbook, "Korean fermented anchovy sauce has softer undertones and is mellower than its Southeast Asian cousins." *Jeotgal* (and other fish sauces for the matter) imparts a rich umami-ness to anything you add it to. You'll have to go to a Korean market to procure *jeotgal*, but the Vietnamese fish sauce Red Boat, found in many supermarkets, is a great alternative and is also made with anchovies.

Fermenting: Fall kimchi is traditionally fermented at lower temperatures (50° to 55°F) for a much longer period. This method favors the heterofermentative *Leuconostoc* bacteria and results in a deeper, richer flavor. This practice goes back to the era when massive amounts of kimchi were "put up" in the fall. The kimchi was packed into traditional Korean fermentation crocks, called *onggi* pots (see page 47), then buried in the ground and fermented at earth temperature during the cold season. This kimchi was a vital source of sustenance during the harsh Korean winters, possibly constituting the only vegetables available until spring arrived. This method required a much longer fermentation time to accomplish the acidification and preservation of the cabbage. Most of us aren't going to go to the trouble of burying a crock in the backyard, however fun it may sound. You can buy specialized kimchi refrigerators to ferment at this lower temperature, but we find that simply fermenting for five days at 64°F also makes delicious kimchi.

TOP USES FOR BRINE FROM KRAUTS, KIMCHI, BRINED FERMENTS, OR PICKLES

Finish sauces and soups: Add brine from any kraut, kimchi, brined ferment, or pickle to brighten flavors with acidity and salt.

Smoothies: Add a shot of natural brine from Basic Kraut (page 92) to a smoothie.

Cocktails: Add a shot of natural brine from Chipotle-Lime Kraut with Cacao (page 110) to a Bloody Mary.

Replace the olive juice in a martini with a shot of natural brine from Basic Kraut (page 92).

Mix 1 part natural brine from George's Bay Kraut (page 112) with 1 part bourbon and 3 parts lemonade for a Pickled Surfer.

Hangover cure: Heat bone broth and coconut milk, stir in a raw egg, remove from the heat, and let cool for 5 minutes. Add a shot of natural brine from kimchi (see pages 128 to 155) or Surf-and-Turf Kraut (page 105).

Salad dressing: Replace half of the vinegar in your favorite dressing recipe with natural brine from any of the krauts.

Brined eggs: Soak hard-boiled eggs in Thymely Beets brine (see page 222) for 2 to 4 days.

Brined French fries: Soak raw potatoes, sliced into fries, in half-sour pickle salt brine (see page 246) for 1 hour before frying.

Brining chicken and pork: Mix enough brine from any kraut, kimchi, brined ferment, or pickle with water at a 1:1 ratio to cover the meat and add 1 tablespoon of salt for every gallon of the liquid mixture. Brine for 6 to 12 hours.

Ceviche: Use a mix of half Taco Bar Mix brine (see page 210) and half fresh lime juice to cure raw seafood.

MAK BAECHU–STYLE KIMCHI

MAKES ½ GALLON

1,400 grams chopped napa cabbage (2-inch square pieces)

260 grams sliced daikon radish (¼-inch-thick half-moons)

100 grams chopped green onions (2-inch-long pieces)

40 grams coarse unrefined sea salt

200 grams Traditional-Style Kimchi Paste (page 130) or California-Style Kimchi Paste (page 131)

2 whole cabbage leaves

EQUIPMENT

Kitchen scale

Latex gloves

½-gallon or 2-liter wide-mouth glass jar

Canning funnel (optional)

Kraut tamper (optional)

Fermentation lid

Fermentation Temperature & Time

Above 68°F
Ferment 3 days or less

65° to 68°F
Ferment 3 to 5 days

Ideal: 64°F
Ferment for 5 days

60° to 63°F
Ferment 5 to 7 days

Below 60°F
Ferment 7 days or more

This style of *baechu* (cabbage) kimchi is known as *mak kimchi—mak* means "simple," and refers to the square cut used for the cabbage. In contrast, for *poggi kimchi*, which is most commonly made in the annual fall tradition of *kimjang* (see "Kraut Fest," page 111), the cabbage is cut in half and brined, then the cabbage halves are stuffed with a seasoning paste and fermented for an extended period during the cold season.

1. Wash and sanitize all your fermentation equipment, including a large bowl, knife, and cutting board, and set aside to air-dry.

2. Put the chopped cabbage, daikon, green onions, and salt in the large bowl. Using gloved hands, vigorously massage, squeeze, and mix the vegetables until they begin to release liquid, about 5 minutes. The cabbage will transform in color and texture, becoming more translucent and pliable as you go. When you can grab a handful of the mixture and squeeze the liquid out of it easily, it's ready to go. Add the kimchi paste and mix it in by hand until well combined.

3. Transfer the mixture to the jar along with the natural brine at the bottom of the bowl (a canning funnel is useful here and helps to minimize spillage). As you add the mixture, tamp it down with your fist or a kraut tamper to submerge the solids under the brine and force out any air pockets. Continue until the jar is almost full, leaving 2 inches of headspace.

4. Take one of the two whole cabbage leaves, give it a quick rinse, and fold it up so it fits into the mouth of the jar. It should cover all the kimchi below and very slightly protrude from the top of the jar. Depending on the size and density of the leaves, you may need to fold and add the second cabbage leaf if the kimchi is not submerged under the brine when the lid is sealed.

5. Seal the jar with the fermentation lid. You should feel some resistance from the cabbage leaf, but not so much that tightening the lid is overly difficult. Place the sealed jar in a bowl to catch any liquid displaced through the airlock during fermentation.

6. Ferment the kimchi in a cool place away from direct sunlight (5 days at 64°F is ideal—see the chart at left). Taste the kimchi after 5 days. When the kimchi is slightly sour but still has some effervescence left (a bite should reveal a burst of bubbly CO_2), it is ready. If it's not sour enough, reseal the jar and let it ferment for another day or two, then taste again. When the kimchi is ready, replace the fermentation lid with a regular lid, seal, and store in the refrigerator for up to 6 months.

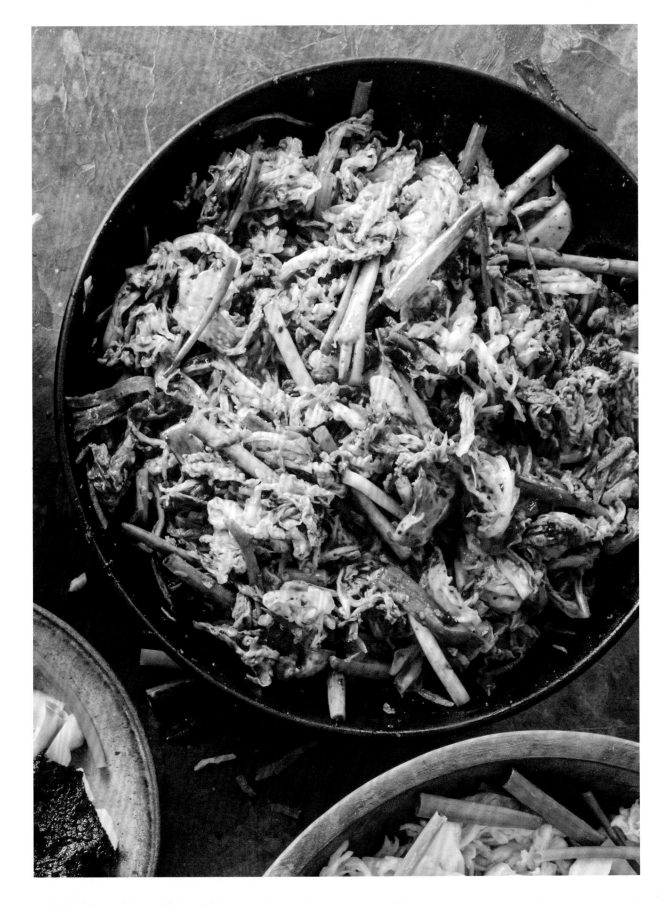

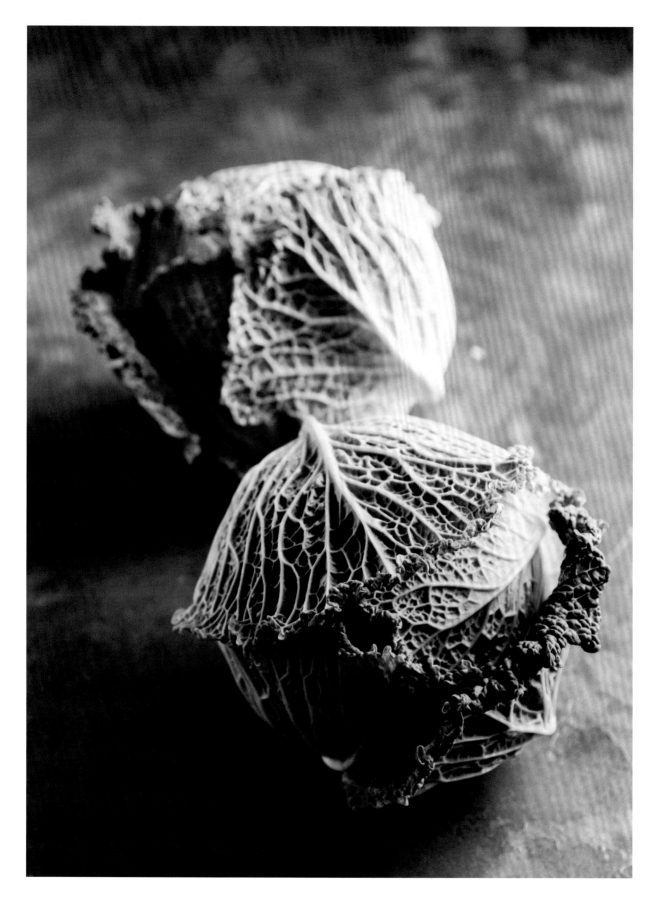

CALIFORNIA KIMCHI
with Savoy Cabbage

MAKES ½ GALLON

1,400 grams chopped savoy cabbage (2-inch square pieces)

120 grams sliced daikon radish (¼-inch-thick half-moons)

120 grams shredded carrots

120 grams chopped green onions (2-inch-long pieces)

40 grams coarse unrefined sea salt

200 grams California-Style Kimchi Paste (page 131) or Traditional-Style Kimchi Paste (page 130)

2 whole cabbage leaves

EQUIPMENT

Kitchen scale

Latex gloves

½-gallon or 2-liter wide-mouth glass jar

Canning funnel (optional)

Kraut tamper (optional)

Fermentation lid

When I decided to make a kimchi for the company, I was a little nervous. Knowing how fiercely protective Koreans are of their beloved ferment, I wanted to make sure I got it right. As I dove into the history of kimchi traditions, my initial hesitancy dissolved. This is a place-based ferment if there ever was one, and the best way I could show reverence would be to emulate that respect for place by creating a California kimchi.

We took the same approach when creating this recipe. Named after the Savoy region in France, savoy cabbage grows abundantly in California. It is an unsung and underutilized brassica that lies somewhere between green and napa cabbage in terms of texture and flavor, and we were itching to use it in kimchi recipe. The result was a tender, flavorful kimchi that we think our Korean friends would approve of—and we think you will, too. You could also substitute whatever cabbage variety grows abundantly near you for more of a localized "kraut-chi." —Kathryn

1. Wash and sanitize all your fermentation equipment, including a large bowl, knife, and cutting board, and set aside to air-dry.

2. Put the chopped cabbage, daikon, carrots, and green onions in the large bowl. Sprinkle the salt over the vegetables. Using gloved hands, vigorously massage, squeeze, and mix the kimchi until the vegetables begin to release liquid, about 5 minutes. The cabbage will transform in color and texture, becoming more translucent and pliable as you go. When you can grab a handful of the mixture and squeeze the liquid out of it easily, it's ready to go. Add the kimchi paste and mix it in by hand until well combined.

3. Transfer the mixture to the jar along with the natural brine at the bottom of the bowl (a canning funnel is useful here and helps to minimize spillage). As you add the mixture, tamp it down with your fist or a kraut tamper to submerge the solids under the brine and force out any air pockets. Continue until the jar is almost full, leaving 2 inches of headspace.

4. Take one of the two whole cabbage leaves, give it a quick rinse, and fold it up so it fits into the mouth of the jar. It should cover all the kimchi below and very slightly protrude from the top

CONTINUED ›

of the jar. Depending on the size and density of the leaves, you may need to fold and add the second cabbage leaf if the kimchi is not submerged under the brine when the lid is sealed.

5. Seal the jar with the fermentation lid. You should feel some resistance from the cabbage leaf, but not so much that tightening the lid is overly difficult. Place the sealed jar on a plate or in a bowl to catch any liquid displaced through the airlock during fermentation.

6. Ferment the kimchi in a cool place away from direct sunlight (5 days at 64°F is ideal—see the chart on page 128). Taste the kimchi after 5 days. When the kimchi is slightly sour but still has some effervescence left (a bite should reveal a burst of bubbly CO_2), it is ready. If it's not sour enough, reseal the jar and let it ferment for another day or two, then taste again. When the kimchi is ready, replace the fermentation lid with a regular lid, seal, and store in the refrigerator for up to 6 months.

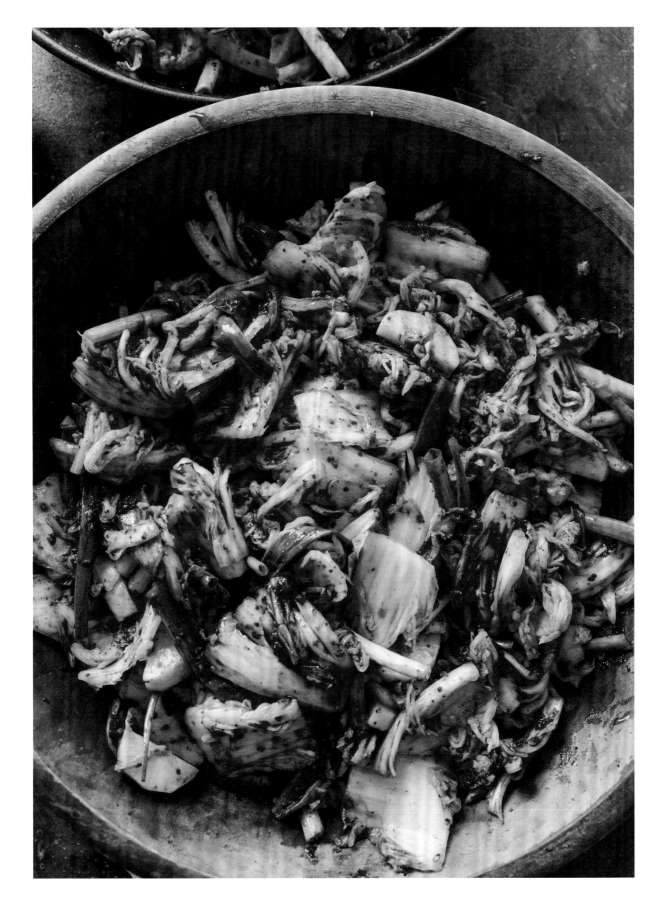

250 milliliters bone broth

30 grams dried mushrooms

1,400 grams chopped napa cabbage (2-inch square pieces)

150 grams sliced daikon radish (¼-inch-thick half-moons)

100 grams chopped green onions (2-inch-long pieces)

30 grams grated or diced peeled fresh ginger

40 grams coarse unrefined sea salt

2 whole cabbage leaves

EQUIPMENT

Kitchen scale

½-gallon or 2-liter wide-mouth glass jar

Canning funnel (optional)

Kraut tamper (optional)

Fermentation lid

WHITE KIMCHI
with Bone Broth and Mushrooms

Shane loves spice, but I'm not a fan of spicy food, so I was delighted to learn there were "white" kimchis. In fact, I was so taken with these milder versions that at one point, we made a "White Girl" Kimchi simply by removing the spicy paste from our California Kimchi, and sold it exclusively at farmers' markets for a summer. The idea to add bone broth and mushrooms started to take shape at the International Kimchi Conference in Washington, DC, where I learned that both are used to create an umami richness in kimchis from the northern region of the Korean peninsula.

Chicken broth and beef broth both work well, and although we have not tried it, we imagine a good vegetable broth would work beautifully, too. We buy local bone broth that is so gelatinous, a spoon will stand up in it when it's cold. The gut-healing properties of the gelatin in bone broth are well documented, making this an exceptionally nutritious kimchi.

Dried mushrooms can be expensive, so feel free to cut back on the quantity, but please don't use fresh mushrooms in this recipe. They are unpredictable and can get downright weird in the crock. At the time of this writing, Costco sells a wonderful blend of dried wild mushrooms for a reasonable price.
—Kathryn

1. Wash and sanitize all your fermentation equipment, including a large bowl, knife, and cutting board, and set aside to air-dry.

2. In a small saucepan, heat the bone broth over medium-high heat until it's just about to boil. Remove from the heat and add the dried mushrooms. Cover and let soak for 20 minutes.

3. Put the chopped cabbage, daikon, green onions, and ginger in the large bowl. Sprinkle the salt over the vegetables. Vigorously massage, squeeze, and mix the kimchi until the vegetables begin to release liquid, about 5 minutes. The cabbage will transform in color and texture, becoming more translucent and pliable as you go. When you can grab a handful of the mixture and squeeze the liquid out of it easily, it's ready to go. Once the bone broth and rehydrated mushrooms have cooled to room temperature, add them to the cabbage mixture and combine.

4. Transfer the mixture to the jar along with the natural brine at the bottom of the bowl (a canning funnel is useful here and helps to minimize spillage). As you add the mixture, tamp it down with your fist or a kraut tamper to submerge the solids under the brine and force out any air pockets. Continue until the jar is almost full, leaving 2 inches of headspace.

5. Take one of the two whole cabbage leaves, give it a quick rinse, and fold it up so it fits into the mouth of the jar. It should cover all the kimchi below and very slightly protrude from the top of the jar. Depending on the size and density of the leaves, you may need to fold and add the second cabbage leaf if the kimchi is not submerged under the brine when the lid is sealed.

6. Seal the jar with the fermentation lid. You should feel some resistance from the cabbage leaf, but not so much that tightening the lid is overly difficult. Place the sealed jar on a plate or in a bowl to catch any liquid displaced through the airlock during fermentation.

7. Ferment the kimchi in a cool place away from direct sunlight (5 days at 64°F is ideal—see the chart on page 128). Taste the kimchi after 5 days. When the kimchi is slightly sour but still has some effervescence left (a bite should reveal a burst of bubbly CO_2), it is ready. If it's not sour enough, reseal the jar and let it ferment for another day or two, then taste again. When the kimchi is ready, replace the fermentation lid with a regular lid, seal, and store in the refrigerator for up to 6 months.

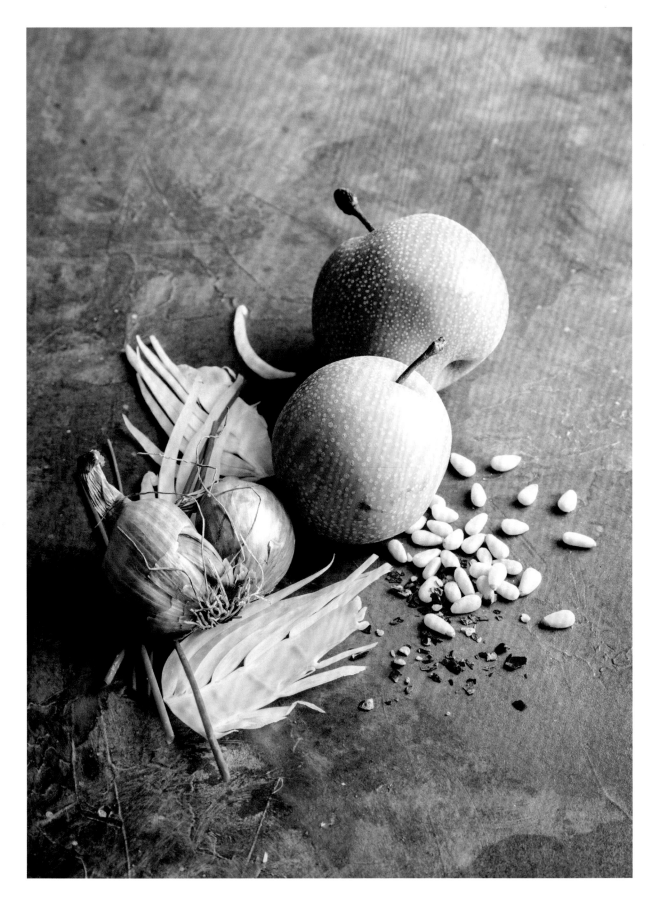

WATER KIMCHI
with Asian Pear and Pine Nuts

MAKES ½ GALLON

960 milliliters filtered water

40 grams coarse unrefined
sea salt

600 grams chopped napa
cabbage (2-inch square pieces)

160 grams sliced Asian pear

100 grams thinly sliced
fennel bulb

80 grams finely diced shallots

30 grams chopped fresh chives
(2-inch pieces)

30 grams pine nuts

½ to 1 teaspoon red pepper
flakes (optional)

2 whole cabbage leaves

EQUIPMENT

Kitchen scale

½-gallon or 2-liter wide-mouth
glass jar

Canning funnel (optional)

Kraut tamper (optional)

Fermentation lid

In 2009, we cheered when our local three-Michelin-starred chef, David Kinch of Manresa, beat Bobby Flay with a quick pear sauerkraut on *Iron Chef America*. The sauerkraut was not fermented but rather made on the fly with vinegar, which allowed the pear flavor to come through. Kinch's ingenuity ignited the idea for this kimchi.

In Korea, pears are commonly used in "water kimchis" (brined kimchis). Much like Kinch's abbreviated sauerkraut, the short fermentation time for kimchi allows the pear essence to shine through the acidity. The pine nuts add a layer of complementary flavor that balances the lightness of the kimchi with a dose of healthy fat. In Korea, this water kimchi is often used as the base for cold soups in the summer, and we've discovered that it's especially tasty served with a dashi broth over cold soba noodles.

If you can't find Asian pears, Boscs are a good alternative, but any firm-fleshed pear will do. Pine nuts can quickly overpower the subtle flavor of the pear, so don't be tempted to add more than we've called for here. We like this kimchi to finish with just a hint of heat, but feel free to omit the red pepper flakes if you prefer a spiceless ferment.

One day, we're going to bring David Kinch a jar of this kimchi, with the recipe and a thank-you note attached.

1. Wash and sanitize all your fermentation equipment, including a large bowl, knife, and cutting board, and set aside to air-dry.

2. Make a brine by bringing 300 milliliters of the water to just under a boil in a small saucepan. Remove from the heat, add the salt, and stir well until all the salt has dissolved. Add the remaining 660 milliliters room-temperature water to the hot brine to cool it down; set aside.

3. Put the chopped cabbage, pear, fennel, shallots, chives, pine nuts, and red pepper flakes in the large bowl. Mix the ingredients until well combined and pack into the jar (a canning funnel is useful here and helps to minimize spillage). You may have to press down with your hand or a kraut tamper to get all the dry ingredients into the jar. Pour the brine into the jar, leaving about 2 inches of headspace.

CONTINUED >

4. Take one of the two whole cabbage leaves, give it a quick rinse, and fold it up so it fits into the mouth of the jar. It should cover all the kimchi below and very slightly protrude from the top of the jar. Depending on the size and density of the leaves, you may need to fold and add the second cabbage leaf if the kimchi is not submerged under the brine when the lid is sealed.

5. Seal the jar with the fermentation lid. You should feel some resistance from the cabbage leaf, but not so much that tightening the lid is overly difficult. Place the sealed jar on a plate or in a bowl to catch any liquid displaced through the airlock during fermentation.

6. Ferment the kimchi in a cool place away from direct sunlight (5 days at 64°F is ideal—see the chart on page 128). Taste the kimchi after 5 days. When the kimchi is slightly sour but still has some effervescence left (a bite should reveal a burst of bubbly CO_2), it is ready. If it's not sour enough, reseal the jar and let it ferment for another day or two, then taste again. When the kimchi is ready, replace the fermentation lid with a regular lid, seal, and store in the refrigerator for up to 6 months.

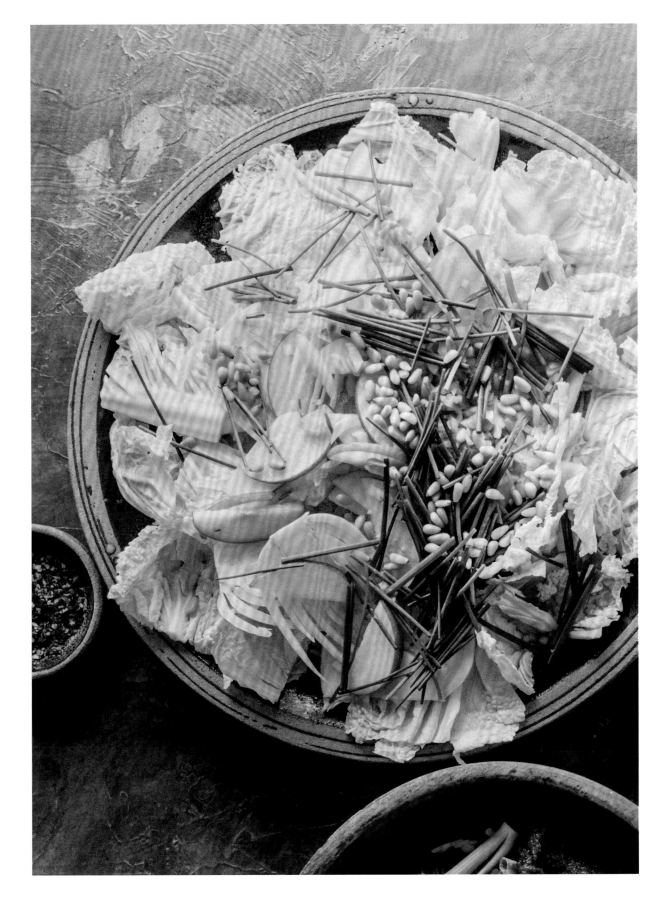

SEAFOOD KIMCHI

DASHI BROTH

200 milliliters filtered water

½ cup bonito flakes, loosely packed

4 pieces kombu seaweed

1,300 grams chopped napa cabbage (2-inch square pieces)

100 grams chopped green onions (2-inch-long pieces)

40 grams coarse unrefined sea salt

200 grams Traditional-Style Kimchi Paste (page 130) or California-Style Kimchi Paste (page 131)

150 grams raw seafood (shucked oysters, baby squid, bay shrimp, or a combination)

2 whole cabbage leaves

EQUIPMENT

Kitchen scale

Latex gloves

Fine-mesh sieve

½-gallon or 2-liter wide-mouth glass jar

Canning funnel (optional)

Kraut tamper (optional)

Fermentation lid

For us Westerners, the idea of putting raw seafood into something that's going to be left at room temperature for a week may sound horrifying, but rest assured, raw oysters and other raw seafood are common additions to kimchi. The acidification of the ferment will essentially "cook" the seafood (much like ceviche is "cooked" by the acids in citrus juice), rendering it safe to eat.

This super-umami-packed kimchi gets its rich sea flavors from nearly every angle. Dashi broth, kimchi paste containing anchovy sauce and salted shrimp, and raw seafood all contribute to this unique, albeit "out-there," ferment. As with any seafood, but especially here, freshness is key and will result in the best flavor. If you are concerned about the freshness of your seafood, then you should not use it, and instead replace the raw seafood portion of this recipe with an additional 150 grams chopped cabbage, or find fresher seafood.

If using raw oysters, make sure you save and include their liquor, that lovely juice that lies within each mollusk. Also, because raw oysters and their liquor are quite salty, it's a good idea to lower the salt by approximately 10 grams (to 30 grams) if you're using oysters only instead of a combination of raw seafood.

1. Wash and sanitize all your fermentation equipment, including a large bowl, knife, and cutting board, and set aside to air-dry.

2. To make the dashi broth, bring the water to a boil in a small saucepan. Remove from the heat and add the bonito flakes and kombu. Cover and let soak for 10 to 15 minutes.

3. Put the chopped cabbage, green onions, and salt in a large bowl. Using gloved hands, vigorously massage, squeeze, and mix the kimchi until the cabbage begins to release liquid, about 5 minutes. The cabbage will transform in color and texture, becoming more translucent and pliable as you go. When you can grab a handful of the mixture and squeeze the liquid out of it easily, it's ready to go.

4. Strain the dashi broth through a fine-mesh sieve into a bowl, pressing down on the solids with your hands or a wooden spoon to extract as much of the liquid as possible; discard the spent solids. Add the dashi broth, kimchi paste, and seafood to the bowl with the vegetables and gently fold them in until combined.

5. Transfer the mixture to the jar along with the natural brine at the bottom of the bowl (a canning funnel is useful here and helps to minimize spillage). As you add the mixture, tamp it down with your fist or a kraut tamper to submerge the solids under the brine and force out any air pockets. Continue until the jar is almost full, leaving 2 inches of headspace.

6. Take one of the two whole cabbage leaves, give it a quick rinse, and fold it up so it fits into the mouth of the jar. It should cover all the kimchi below and very slightly protrude from the top of the jar. Depending on the size and density of the leaves, you may need to fold and add the second cabbage leaf if the kimchi is not submerged under the brine when the lid is sealed.

7. Seal the jar with the fermentation lid. You should feel some resistance from the cabbage leaf, but not so much that tightening the lid is overly difficult. Place the sealed jar on a plate or in a bowl to catch any liquid displaced through the airlock during fermentation.

8. Ferment the kimchi in a cool place away from direct sunlight (7 days at 64°F is ideal—see the chart at right). Because this recipe contains raw seafood, we advise you to ferment it longer than the other kimchis to ensure that the seafood gets fully acidified. Taste the kimchi after 7 days. When the kimchi is slightly sour but still has some effervescence left (a bite should reveal a burst of bubbly CO_2), it is ready. If it's not sour enough, reseal the jar and let it ferment for another day or two, then taste again. When the kimchi is ready, replace the fermentation lid with a regular lid, seal, and store in the refrigerator for up to 3 months.

Fermentation
Temperature & Time

Above 68°F
Ferment 5 days or less

65° to 68°F
Ferment 5 to 7 days

Ideal: 64°F
Ferment 7 days

60° to 63°F
Ferment 7 to 10 days

Below 60°F
Ferment 10 days or more

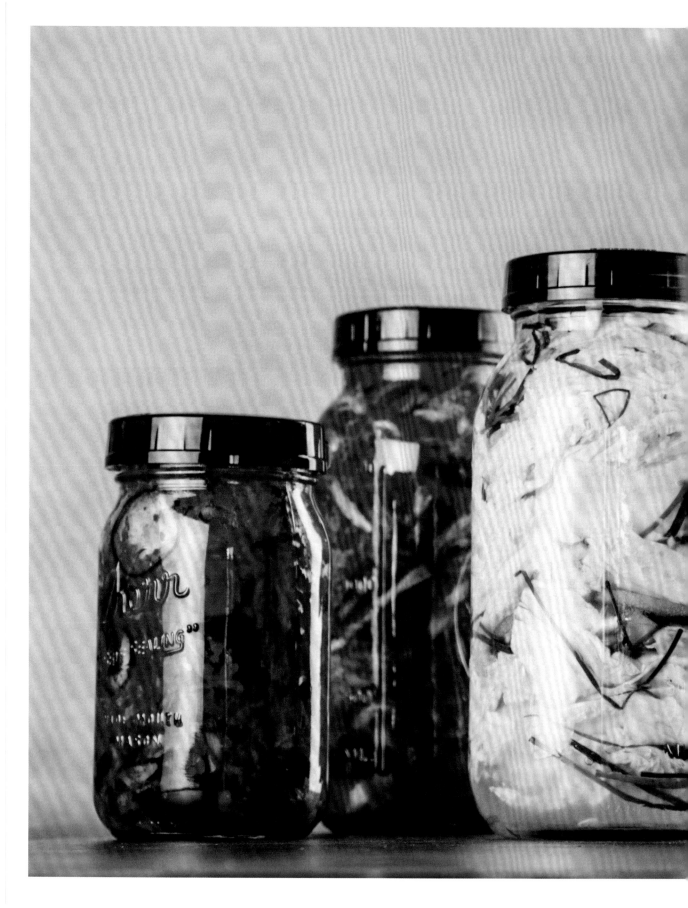

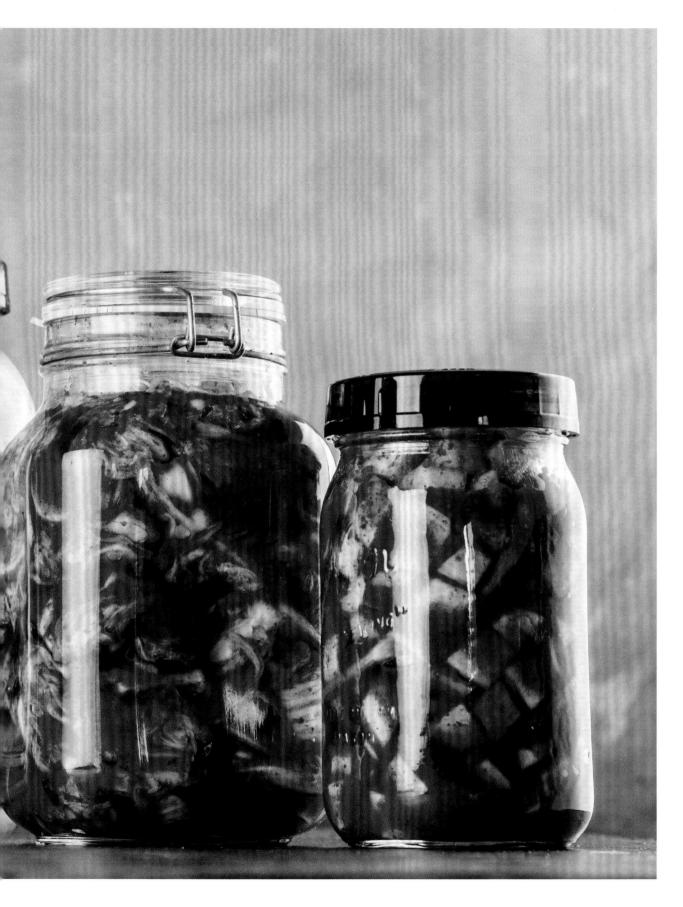

MAKES 1 QUART

760 grams sliced peeled
kabocha squash (1-inch-thick
half-moons; from 1 medium
squash)

20 grams coarse unrefined
sea salt

50 grams coarsely chopped
green onions

100 grams Traditional-Style
Kimchi Paste (page 130) or
California-Style Kimchi Paste
(page 131)

40 grams sprouted hulled
pumpkin seeds

1 round slice of squash (1-inch
thick) that fits into the jar
snuggly, or a glass weight

EQUIPMENT

Kitchen scale

Latex gloves

1-quart or 1-liter wide-mouth
glass jar

Canning funnel (optional)

Kraut tamper (optional)

Fermentation lid

KABOCHA SQUASH KIMCHI
with Pumpkin Seeds

Until a few years ago, most of us had never heard of kabocha squash, but they seem to be everywhere these days. And for good reason—they are incredibly flavorful and a tad sweeter than butternut squash (which, by the way, can stand in as an excellent substitute for kabocha in this recipe). The heat from the kimchi paste is accentuated by the acidity formed during fermentation, and the two come together to provide a beautiful balance to the sweetness of the squash.

The key to making successful winter squash kimchi is making sure the squash is cut small enough that it will soften during the short fermentation time. Slices are better than cubes.

It may seem silly to mix the seeds of one squash with another type of squash, but we just love the flavor and texture of pumpkin seeds in this recipe. Of course, you can use any type of pumpkin seed, including roasted, but if you can find them, raw sprouted seeds up the "healthy" level by making more of their protein, enzymes, and minerals available.

The orange-red hues of this kimchi are stunning against the backdrop of black rice (also known as Forbidden Rice). Drizzled with a tiny bit of dark sesame oil and topped with fresh cilantro, this has become a treasured winter meal.

1. Wash and sanitize all your fermentation equipment, including a large bowl, knife, and cutting board, and set aside to air-dry.

2. In the large bowl, toss the squash with the salt. Add the green onions and toss to combine. Add the kimchi paste and the pumpkin seeds. Using gloved hands, gently mix the kimchi until the squash begins to release liquid, about 5 minutes. The squash won't release lots of juice like cabbage does, but it will release some.

3. Transfer the kimchi to the jar (a canning funnel is useful here and helps to minimize spillage). As you add the kimchi, tamp it down with your fist or a kraut tamper to submerge the solids under the brine and force out any air pockets. Continue until the jar is almost full, leaving 2 inches of headspace.

4. Take the 1-inch-thick squash piece and place it into the mouth of the jar. It should cover most of the vegetables below and very slightly protrude from the top of the jar.

5. Seal the jar with the fermentation lid. Place the sealed jar on a plate or in a bowl to catch any liquid displaced through the airlock during fermentation.

6. Ferment the kimchi in a cool place away from direct sunlight (5 days at 64°F is ideal—see the chart on page 128). Taste the kimchi after 5 days to determine if the flavor and sourness are to your liking. If it's not sour enough, reseal the jar and let it ferment for another day or two, then taste again. When the kimchi is ready, replace the fermentation lid with a regular lid, seal, and store in the refrigerator for up to 6 months.

DAIKON RADISH KIMCHI

MAKES 1 QUART

800 grams diced daikon radish
(½-inch cubes)

50 grams chopped green onions
(2-inch-long pieces)

20 grams coarse unrefined
sea salt

100 grams Traditional-Style
Kimchi Paste (page 130) or
California-Style Kimchi Paste
(page 131)

1 slice of daikon radish (1-inch
thick) that fits into the jar
snuggly, or a glass weight

EQUIPMENT

Kitchen scale

Latex gloves

1-quart or 1-liter wide-mouth
glass jar

Canning funnel (optional)

Kraut tamper (optional)

Fermentation lid

Many years ago, when I was studying macrobiotic cooking in Brazil, I tasted my first fermented daikon radish and became a forever fan. The deliciously mellow, salty tuber had been fermented using a Japanese technique called *nukazuke*. Although this method is very different than the one used for this kimchi ferment, lactobacilli figures prominently in both, which produces a more acidic flavor profile.

The Korean radishes, or *mu*, typically used in kimchi can be hard to find outside Korean markets, so we use daikon radishes, which are readily available in supermarkets everywhere. Younger, smaller daikons are milder and more tender, which we prefer. You'll want to give them a good scrub to remove any dirt stuck in the crevices, but don't peel them, as the lactic acid bacteria on the skin is important to the success and flavor of this ferment.

Radish kimchi is one of our favorite noncabbage versions and is excellent eaten with rice or tossed into a stir-fry at the last minute (to preserve the microbes). —Kathryn

1. Wash and sanitize all your fermentation equipment, including a large bowl, knife, and cutting board, and set aside to air-dry.

2. In the large bowl, combine the chopped daikon and the green onions. Sprinkle the salt over the vegetables. Add the kimchi paste. Using gloved hands, thoroughly mix the kimchi until the daikon begins to release liquid, about 5 minutes. The daikon won't release lots of juice like cabbage does, but it will release some.

3. Transfer the mixture to the jar along with the natural brine at the bottom of the bowl (a canning funnel is useful here and helps to minimize spillage). As you add the mixture, tamp it down with your fist or a kraut tamper to submerge the solids under the brine and force out any air pockets. Continue until the jar is almost full, leaving 2 inches of headspace.

4. Take the 1-inch-thick daikon slice and place it into the mouth of the jar. It should cover most of the vegetables below and very slightly protrude from the top of the jar.

5. Seal the jar with the fermentation lid. You should feel some resistance from the daikon slice, but not so much that tightening the lid is overly difficult. Place the sealed jar on a plate or in a bowl to catch any liquid displaced through the airlock during fermentation.

6. Ferment the kimchi in a cool place away from direct sunlight (5 days at 64°F is ideal—see the chart on page 128). Taste the kimchi after 5 days. When the kimchi is slightly sour but still has some effervescence left (a bite should reveal a burst of bubbly CO_2), it is ready. If it's not sour enough, reseal the jar and let it ferment for another day or two, then taste again. When the kimchi is ready, replace the fermentation lid with a regular lid, seal, and store in the refrigerator for up to 6 months.

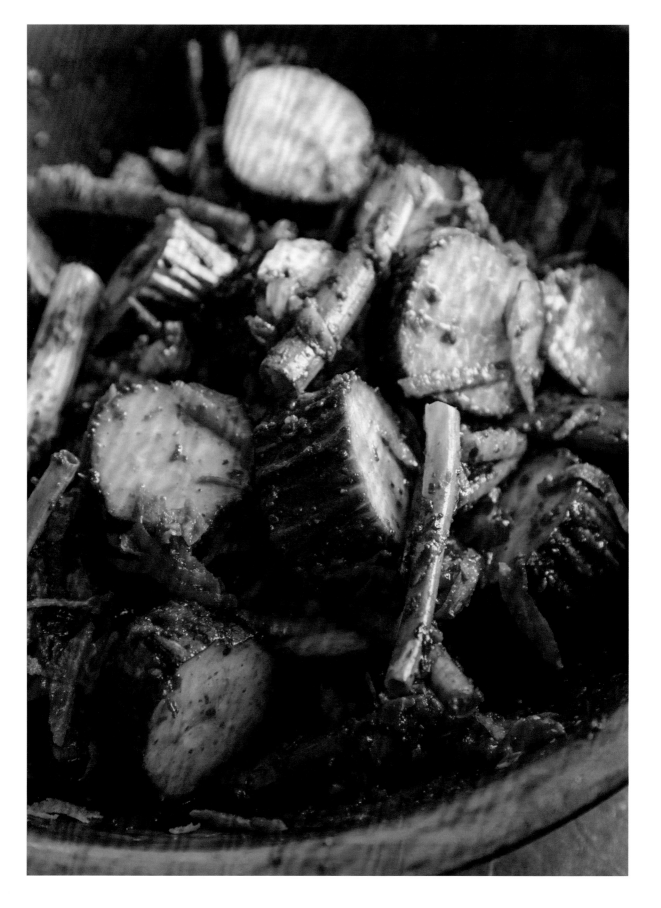

CUCUMBER KIMCHI

MAKES 1 QUART

700 grams sliced cucumbers
(1-inch-thick half-moons)

20 grams coarse unrefined
sea salt

100 grams shredded carrots

50 grams chopped green onions
(2-inch-long pieces)

100 grams Traditional-Style
Kimchi Paste (page 130) or
California-Style Kimchi Paste
(page 131)

EQUIPMENT

Kitchen scale

Latex gloves

1-quart or 1-liter wide-mouth
glass jar

Canning funnel (optional)

Kraut tamper (optional)

Glass weight or other type
of weight

Fermentation lid

We've been making this kimchi "pickle" for a number of years and we never tire of it. Although it's traditionally a summer ferment, we eat this kimchi year-round. Traditionally, the cucumber is cut into quarters with the bottom end left intact, which allows the cucumber to be "stuffed" with kimchi paste. You can certainly do this, but we find a simpler cut preferable. Not only does it make preparation easier, but it's nice to be able to pull out a bite-size chunk rather than having to take the whole cucumber out of the jar just to pull off a piece.

Persian or English hothouse cucumbers, commonly called "slicers," have soft skins and relatively few seeds, which make them ideal for a short, dry-salt ferment like this one. We have a slight preference for Persians because of their smaller size and the fact that they don't come wrapped in plastic like English cucumbers. Avoid pickling cucumbers like Kirbys, as their thicker, tannic skins are better suited to brining. If you have access, a number of other varieties, like plump, yellow-skinned Armenian cucumbers, work equally well.

If you're growing your own cucumbers, pick them long before they get too big or start to go to seed, and if you're buying them at the store, make sure to select the freshest ones possible. Don't peel the cucumbers—just give them a rinse to remove any dirt. An enzyme from the flowering end of the cucumber can cause pickles to soften, so when you're prepping them, take special care to ensure the ends and any attached flowers have been removed and don't make their way into the kimchi.

These kimchi cucumbers are divine right out of the jar, but you can also enjoy them unfermented—they make a delicious addition to a salad or with a dish like *bibimbap*, made of rice, fresh and fermented vegetables, and topped with a fried egg. To make a fresh, unfermented version to be eaten right away, thinly slice the cucumbers and mix them with the paste and half of the salt. Taste after mixing and adjust the salt to taste. Let the mixture sit for 15 to 30 minutes, allowing the cucumbers to release a bit of liquid, then mix again and serve.

CONTINUED ›

1. Wash and sanitize all your fermentation equipment, including a large bowl, knife, and cutting board, and set aside to air-dry.

2. Put the cucumbers in the large bowl. Add the salt and gently massage for about 1 minute (this will help the cucumbers render their liquid). Add the carrots and the green onions to the bowl with the cucumbers and toss to combine. Add the kimchi paste. Using gloved hands, gently mix the kimchi until the vegetables begin to release liquid, about 5 minutes.

3. Transfer the mixture to the jar along with the natural brine at the bottom of the bowl (a canning funnel is useful here and helps to minimize spillage). As you add the mixture, tamp it down with your fist or a kraut tamper to submerge the solids under the brine and force out any air pockets. Continue until the jar is almost full, leaving 2 inches of headspace.

4. Add the weight of your choice to the top of the ferment. The weight should cover all of the vegetables below and slightly protrude from the jar.

5. Seal the jar with the fermentation lid. You should feel some resistance from the weight, but not so much that tightening the lid is overly difficult. Place the sealed jar on a plate or in a bowl to catch any liquid displaced through the airlock during fermentation.

6. Ferment the kimchi in a cool place away from direct sunlight (5 days at 64°F is ideal—see the chart on page 128). Taste the kimchi after 5 days. When the kimchi is slightly sour but still has some effervescence left (a bite should reveal a burst of bubbly CO_2), it is ready. If it's not sour enough, reseal the jar and let it ferment for another day or two, then taste again. When the kimchi is ready, replace the fermentation lid with a regular lid, seal, and store in the refrigerator for up to 6 months. Cucumbers have a tendency to soften, so be sure to transfer the kimchi to the refrigerator while it still retains its crunch.

CARROT KIMCHI
with Raisins

MAKES 1 QUART

775 grams shredded unpeeled carrots

25 grams raisins

20 grams coarse unrefined sea salt

50 grams coarsely chopped green onions

100 grams Traditional-Style Kimchi Paste (page 130) or California-Style Kimchi Paste (page 131)

EQUIPMENT

Kitchen scale

Latex gloves

1-quart or 1-liter wide-mouth glass jar

Canning funnel (optional)

Kraut tamper (optional)

Glass weight or other type of weight

Fermentation lid

Sometimes the process of elimination yields wonderful recipes. When we realized our fermented carrot slaw (minus the mayo) was a bust, we tried making a kimchi with it, and a star was born.

Don't peel the carrots, but do give them a good rinse. The lactic acid bacteria on their skin is an integral part of making a successful and flavorful ferment. Older carrot skins can become slightly bitter, so use fresh carrots, and because you're not peeling them, make sure they're organic, of course.

1. Wash and sanitize all your fermentation equipment, including a medium bowl, knife, and cutting board, and set aside to air-dry.

2. In the medium bowl, combine the carrots, raisins, and salt and gently massage for about 1 minute. Add the green onions and mix with your hands to combine with the carrots. Add the kimchi paste. Using gloved hands, gently mix the kimchi until the carrots begin to release liquid, about 5 minutes. The carrots won't release lots of juice like cabbage does, but they will release some.

3. Transfer the kimchi to the jar (a canning funnel is useful here and helps to minimize spillage). As you add the mixture, tamp it down with your fist or a kraut tamper to submerge the solids under the brine and to force out any air pockets. Continue until the jar is almost full, leaving 2 inches of headspace.

4. Place the weight in the jar on top of the ferment. The weight should cover all of the vegetables below and slightly protrude from the jar.

5. Seal the jar with the fermentation lid. You should feel some resistance from the weight, but not so much that tightening the lid is overly difficult. Place the sealed jar in a bowl to catch any liquid displaced through the airlock during fermentation.

6. Ferment the kimchi in a cool place away from direct sunlight (5 days at 64°F is ideal—see the chart on page 128). Taste the kimchi after 5 days to determine if the flavor and sourness is are to your liking. If it's not sour enough, reseal the jar and let it ferment for another day or two, then taste again. When the kimchi is ready, replace the fermentation lid with a regular lid, seal, and store in the refrigerator for up to 6 months.

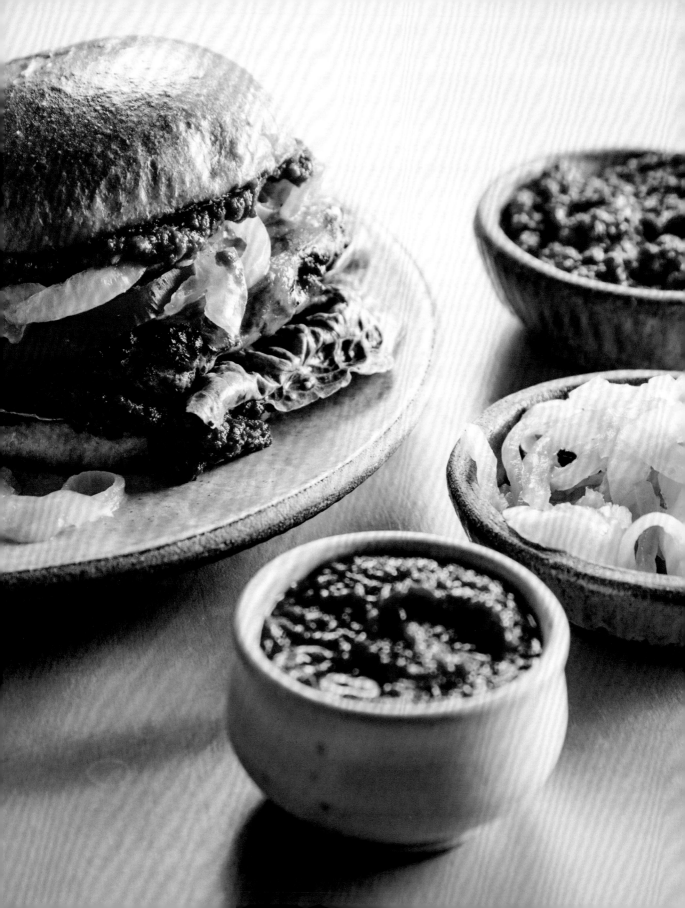

Dry-Salted Ferments

Dry-salting is a very effective method used to extract moisture from vegetables. The juicy "brine" that forms is an ideal environment for the fermentation of a variety of vegetables. Sauerkraut is the most well-known dry-salted ferment, but any number of vegetables ferment beautifully with this method. In fact, the list is so exhaustive, we had a hard time narrowing down which recipes to share with you. (Dry-salt fermenting is not appropriate for *all* vegetables, as a certain level of juiciness is required. Vegetables that are on the drier side are better suited to brining—see page 206.)

A couple of the recipes don't technically fit in this category but they found their way here for one reason or another. The ketchup, for instance is a dry-salt ferment, but tomatoes are a fruit and really belong in the fruit section. That's the last place you'd probably go looking for ketchup, though, so it landed here.

There are a couple of tricks, explained in the Fermenter's Notes, that will help your ferments be the best they can be, but for the most part, dry-salting is the easiest of all ferments and a great place to start if you're new to fermenting.

FERMENTER'S NOTES

Salt: You can use any salt to make the following dry-salted ferments, but a coarse-grained salt is optimal. When it is massaged into the vegetables, it helps to break down the vegetable's cell walls, causing it to release its liquid faster.

The accepted range of salt for dry-salted ferments is 1.5 to 2.5% by weight. All our dry-salted recipes contain 2% salt by weight, which we have found consistently yields superior flavor and crunch. In warmer temperatures, which favor the growth of yeast, the salt can be increased to as high as 2.5% to slow down the fermentation process and favor lactic acid bacteria (LAB). Conversely, if fermenting in cold temperatures, which can slow fermentation time, the salt can be decreased to as low as 1.5% to speed up fermentation. Lower salt content and fermenting at lower temperatures both favor heterofermentative bacteria, resulting in a more flavorful ferment.

Brine: There may be times when you need to make supplemental or replacement brine for your ferment. If your vegetables do not initially produce enough liquid to fully submerge the vegetables, you can make extra brine to top it off—in most cases, 100 grams of brine should be enough. Simply dissolve 2 grams salt in 98 milliliters filtered water and fill the jar with the brine, leaving 2 inches of headspace. This brine can also be used if you lose some of the brine through the airlock or lid during the fermentation process. If this happens, open the jar, add the replacement brine, again leaving 2 inches of headspace, and reseal (leave the jar open only as long as it takes to add the brine, to avoid introducing unwanted yeasts and molds). During the first five to seven days, gas (CO_2) is produced, which can cause the brine to be expelled through the airlock, potentially dropping the brine level below the vegetables. If you add replacement brine too soon, it will just be expelled by the gases too, so wait until the end of this first phase before adding more brine. The exposed vegetables are protected by a layer of CO_2 during this phase and generally will not deteriorate. You'll know this phase is complete when the airlock stops bubbling.

GINGER CARROTS
with Black Sesame

MAKES 1 QUART

900 grams shredded carrots

30 grams grated peeled fresh ginger

20 grams coarse unrefined sea salt

15 grams black sesame seeds

50 milliliters natural brine from Basic Kraut (page 92) or 50 grams Basic Kraut

EQUIPMENT

Kitchen scale

1-quart or 1-liter wide-mouth glass jar

Canning funnel (optional)

Kraut tamper (optional)

Weight

Fermentation lid

Fermentation Temperature & Time

Above 68°F
Ferment 2 weeks or less

65° to 68°F
Ferment 2 to 3 weeks

Ideal: 64°F
Ferment 3 weeks

60° to 63°F
Ferment 3 to 4 weeks

Below 60°F
Ferment 4 weeks or more

For some reason, carrot ferments are hit or miss. We've found that the addition of ginger significantly increases the odds of a successful fermentation, and because the two ingredients pair so well, we now sneak ginger into all our carrot recipes. In this recipe, however, ginger is front and center—no sneaking here.

You might not think carrots would be a good candidate for dry-salting, but if left to hang out with the salt long enough, they do eventually produce enough liquid.

This ferment makes a lovely addition to salads, is great as a topper for Asian-style rice dishes or used in sushi rolls, and, with a little sesame oil, becomes a delightful slaw.

1. Wash and sanitize all your fermentation equipment, including a medium bowl, knife, and cutting board, and set aside to air-dry.

2. In the medium bowl, combine the carrots, ginger, salt, sesame seeds, and kraut brine. Using your hands, massage, squeeze, and mix the carrot mixture until the carrots begin to release liquid, about 5 minutes. When you can grab a handful of shredded carrots and squeeze the liquid out of it easily, it's ready to go.

3. Transfer the carrots to the jar (a canning funnel is useful here and helps to minimize spillage). As you add the carrots, tamp them down with your fist or a kraut tamper to submerge the solids under the brine and force out any air pockets. Continue until the jar is almost full, leaving 1 to 2 inches of headspace.

4. Place the weight in the jar on top of the carrots and press down until the carrots are completely submerged in the brine. Seal the jar with the fermentation lid. Place the sealed jar in a bowl to catch any liquid displaced through the airlock during fermentation.

5. Ferment the carrots in a cool place away from direct sunlight (3 weeks at 64°F is ideal—see the chart at left). Taste the carrots after 2 weeks to determine if the flavor and sourness are to your liking. If they're not sour enough, reseal the jar and let them ferment for another week, then taste again. When the carrots are sour to your liking, replace the fermentation lid with a regular lid, seal, and store in the refrigerator for up to 10 months.

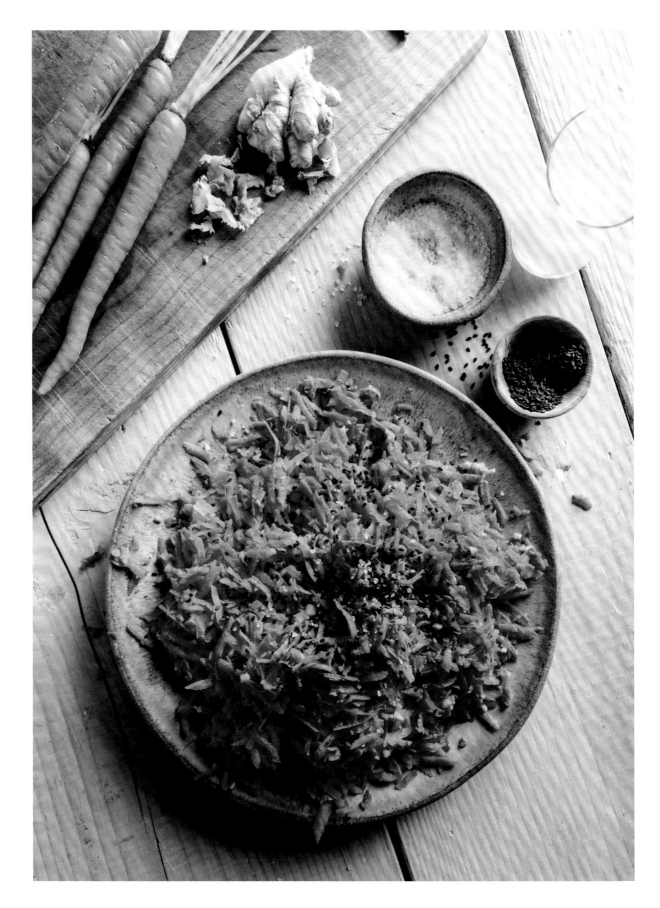

CURRIED DAIKON

850 grams sliced daikon radish (¼-inch-thick half-moons)

50 grams chopped green onions (1-inch pieces)

20 grams coarse unrefined sea salt

20 grams curry powder

50 milliliters natural brine from Basic Kraut (page 92) or 50 grams Basic Kraut

EQUIPMENT

Kitchen scale

Latex gloves

1-quart or 1-liter wide-mouth glass jar

Canning funnel (optional)

Kraut tamper (optional)

Weight

Fermentation lid

We love how fermentation mellows and softens daikon radishes, and they seem to pair particularly well with curry spices. Ditto with green onions, which we like to cut into segments large enough to pull out of the jar and munch on. Muchi curry powder, with its extra cardamom and clove, is a favorite in our kitchen, but any curry works well in this truly scrumptious ferment. Curry powder will stain your hands, so you'll want to wear gloves. This is a gorgeous addition to a vegetable or crudité platter and is wonderful in salads.

1. Wash and sanitize all your fermentation equipment, including a medium bowl, knife, and cutting board, and set aside to air-dry.

2. In the medium bowl, combine the daikon, green onions, salt, curry powder, and kraut brine. Using gloved hands, gently massage, squeeze, and mix the daikon mixture until the daikon begins to release liquid, 3 to 5 minutes. When you can grab a handful of the daikon and squeeze the liquid out of it easily, it's ready to go.

3. Transfer the mixture to the jar (a canning funnel is useful here and helps to minimize spillage). As you add the mixture, tamp it down with your fist or a kraut tamper to submerge the solids under the brine and force out any air pockets. Continue until the jar is almost full, leaving 1 to 2 inches of headspace.

4. Place the weight in the jar on top of the daikon and press down until the daikon is completely submerged in the brine. Seal the jar with the fermentation lid. Place the sealed jar on a plate or in a bowl to catch any liquid displaced through the airlock during fermentation.

5. Ferment the daikon in a cool place away from direct sunlight (3 weeks at 64°F is ideal—see the chart on page 160). Taste the daikon after 2 weeks to determine if the flavor and sourness are to your liking. If it's not sour enough, reseal the jar and let it ferment for another week, then taste again. When the daikon is sour to your liking, replace the fermentation lid with a regular lid, seal, and store in the refrigerator for up to 10 months.

GARDEN SLAW

MAKES 1 QUART

300 grams sliced red radishes
(¼-inch-thick rounds)

300 grams shredded carrots

300 grams sliced peeled
slicing cucumber, such as
Persian or English (¼-inch-
thick half-moons)

20 grams coarse unrefined
sea salt

3 tablespoons coarsely chopped
fresh flat-leaf parsley leaves

3 tablespoons coarsely chopped
fresh cilantro (stems included)

50 milliliters natural brine
from Basic Kraut (page 92)
or 50 grams Basic Kraut

EQUIPMENT

Kitchen scale

1-quart or 1-liter wide-mouth
glass jar

Canning funnel (optional)

Kraut tamper (optional)

Weight

Fermentation lid

This simple and satisfying ferment couldn't be easier to make. Since we have the food processor out, we typically double the vegetables so we can serve half fresh for lunch that day, seasoned with salt to our liking, and ferment the other half, salted according to the recipe, for later. You can use any variety of vegetables in this recipe. Jicama, purple cabbage, green onions, beets, and turnips are just a handful of the many vegetables we've experimented with that work really well here. We like an assortment of vegetable shapes for the visual effect, but you can cut them anyway you like. This is a great recipe to play with and customize into your signature slaw.

One of our favorite ways to eat this slaw is mixed with a handful of fresh herbs and tossed with a little olive oil and then served in a salad bowl.

1. Wash and sanitize all your fermentation equipment, including a medium bowl, knife, and cutting board, and set aside to air-dry.

2. In the medium bowl, combine the radishes, carrots, cucumber, salt, parsley, cilantro, and kraut brine. Using your hands, massage, squeeze, and mix the vegetables until they begin to release liquid, about 5 minutes. When you can grab a handful of slaw and squeeze the liquid out of it easily, it's ready to go.

3. Transfer the slaw to the jar (a canning funnel is useful here and helps to minimize spillage). As you add the slaw, tamp it down with your fist or a kraut tamper to submerge the solids under the brine and force out any air pockets. Continue until the jar is almost full, leaving 1 to 2 inches of headspace.

4. Place the weight in the jar on top of the slaw and press down until the slaw is completely submerged in the brine. Seal the jar with the fermentation lid. Place the sealed jar on a plate or in a bowl to catch any liquid displaced through the airlock during fermentation.

5. Ferment the slaw in a cool place away from direct sunlight (3 weeks at 64°F is ideal—see the chart on page 160). Taste the slaw after 2 weeks to determine if the flavor and sourness are to your liking. If it's not sour enough, reseal the jar and let it ferment for another week, then taste again. When the slaw is sour to your liking, replace the fermentation lid with a regular lid, seal, and store in the refrigerator for up to 10 months.

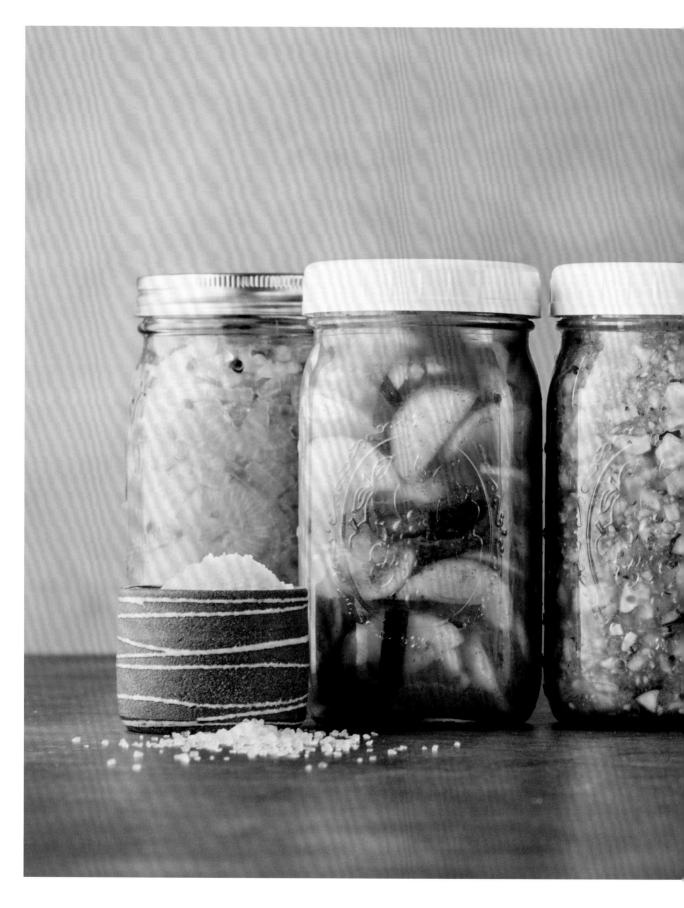

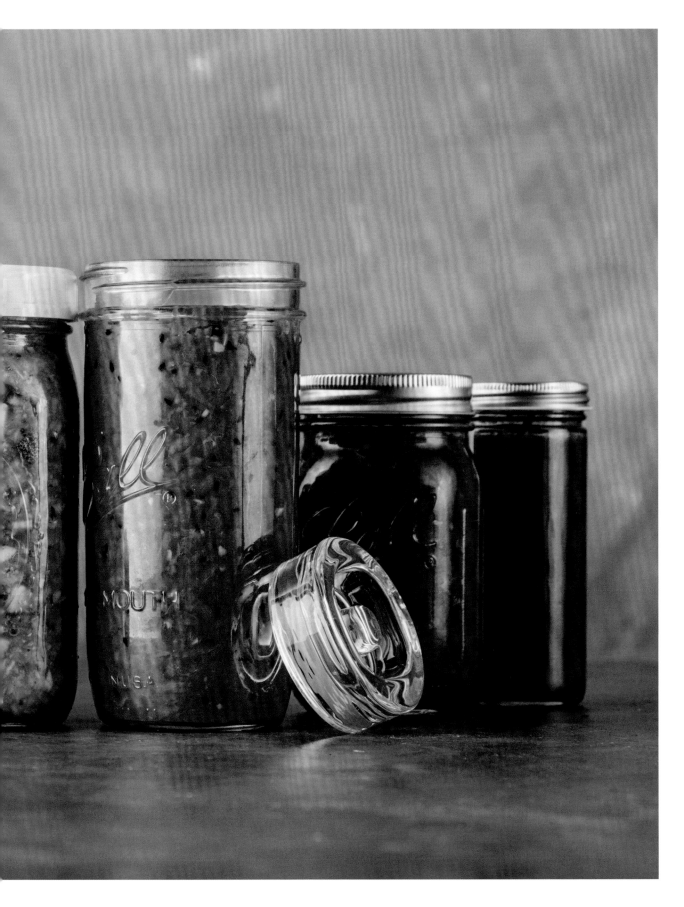

WHEEZY'S CHOWCHOW

600 grams roughly chopped green tomatoes

200 grams coarsely chopped red bell peppers

100 grams coarsely chopped onions

20 grams coarse unrefined sea salt

1 teaspoon yellow mustard seeds

1 teaspoon ground turmeric

½ teaspoon red pepper flakes

¼ teaspoon freshly grated nutmeg

¼ teaspoon ground allspice

¼ teaspoon ground cinnamon

Pinch of ground cloves

50 milliliters natural brine from Basic Kraut (page 92) or 50 grams Basic Kraut

EQUIPMENT

Kitchen scale

1-quart or 1-liter wide-mouth glass jar

Canning funnel (optional)

Kraut tamper (optional)

Weight

Fermentation lid

My grandmother, Louise, whom I affectionately called Wheezy, was a fabulous home cook and an amazing woman. Cut from the cloth of a different era, when everything was homemade, Wheezy loved to cook, bake, can, and preserve and I have countless fond memories of time spent with her in her kitchen. I've adapted this chochow from her original vinegar-based recipe, which she canned in large batches using the leftover green tomatoes from my grandfather Jack's garden. I've included this recipe to pay homage to the woman who partly raised me, and whom I adored. This one's for you, Wheezy. —Shane

1. Wash and sanitize all your fermentation equipment, including a medium bowl, knife, and cutting board, and set aside to air-dry.

2. In the medium bowl, combine the green tomatoes, bell peppers, onion, salt, mustard seeds, turmeric, red pepper flakes, nutmeg, allspice, cinnamon, cloves, and kraut brine. Using your hands, massage, squeeze, and mix the chowchow until the vegetables begin to release liquid, about 5 minutes. When you can grab a handful of vegetables and squeeze the liquid out of it easily, it's ready to go.

3. Transfer the chowchow to the jar along with any liquid (a canning funnel is useful here and helps to minimize spillage). As you add the mixture, tamp it down with your fist or a kraut tamper to submerge the solids under the brine and force out any air pockets. Continue until the jar is almost full, leaving 1 to 2 inches of headspace.

4. Place the weight in the jar on top of the chowchow and press down until the chowchow is completely submerged in the brine. Seal the jar with the fermentation lid. Place the sealed jar on a plate or in a bowl to catch any liquid displaced through the airlock during fermentation.

5. Ferment the chowchow in a cool place away from direct sunlight (3 weeks at 64°F is ideal—see the chart on page 160). Taste the chowchow after 2 weeks to determine if the flavor and sourness are to your liking. If it's not sour enough, reseal the jar and let it ferment for another week, then taste again. When the chowchow is sour to your liking, replace the fermentation lid with a regular lid, seal, and store in the refrigerator for up to 10 months.

TURMERIC–BLACK PEPPER PASTE

MAKES 1 PINT

450 grams coarsely chopped peeled fresh turmeric

1 teaspoon freshly ground black pepper

10 grams coarse unrefined sea salt

25 milliliters natural brine from Basic Kraut (page 92)

EQUIPMENT

Kitchen scale

Food processor or blender

1-pint or ½-liter wide-mouth glass jar

Canning funnel (optional)

Parchment paper or cheesecloth cut to the diameter of the jar

Fermentation lid

Turmeric's active compound, curcumin, has been extensively studied for its disease-fighting potential and preventive health benefits, but it is perhaps best known for its powerful anti-inflammatory properties.

It is worth doing a little research to find turmeric grown locally, because there is a world of difference between freshly harvested turmeric and stuff that's been sitting around, sometimes for months. Fresh turmeric produces significantly more juice, which comes in handy for a dry-salt ferment. Your local co-op or natural grocer will know what's available in your area, and they are generally very happy to order it fresh for you.

Use a little of the paste mixed into coconut milk with a dash of cinnamon and a tiny bit of honey or stevia for a wonderful nighttime tonic. It's also great in smoothies, salad dressings, stir-fries, and, of course, curries.

1. Wash and sanitize all your fermentation equipment, including a knife and cutting board, and set aside to air-dry.

2. Combine the turmeric, pepper, salt, and kraut brine in the food processor and process until the mixture is smooth. Scrape down the sides of the processor bowl with a spatula and process again, until very smooth and well blended.

3. Transfer the turmeric paste to the jar along with any liquid (a canning funnel is useful here and helps to minimize spillage). As you add the mixture, tamp it down with your fist to submerge the solids under the brine and force out any air pockets.

4. Place the parchment paper or cheesecloth in the jar over the turmeric paste (the paste should be completely covered). Seal the jar with the fermentation lid. Place the sealed jar on a plate or in a bowl to catch any liquid displaced through the airlock during fermentation.

5. Ferment the turmeric paste in a cool place away from direct sunlight (3 weeks at 64°F is ideal—see the chart on page 160). Taste the paste after 2 weeks to determine if the flavor and sourness are to your liking. If it's not sour enough, reseal the jar and let it ferment for another week, then taste again. When the paste is sour to your liking, replace the fermentation lid with a regular lid, seal, and store in the refrigerator for up to 10 months.

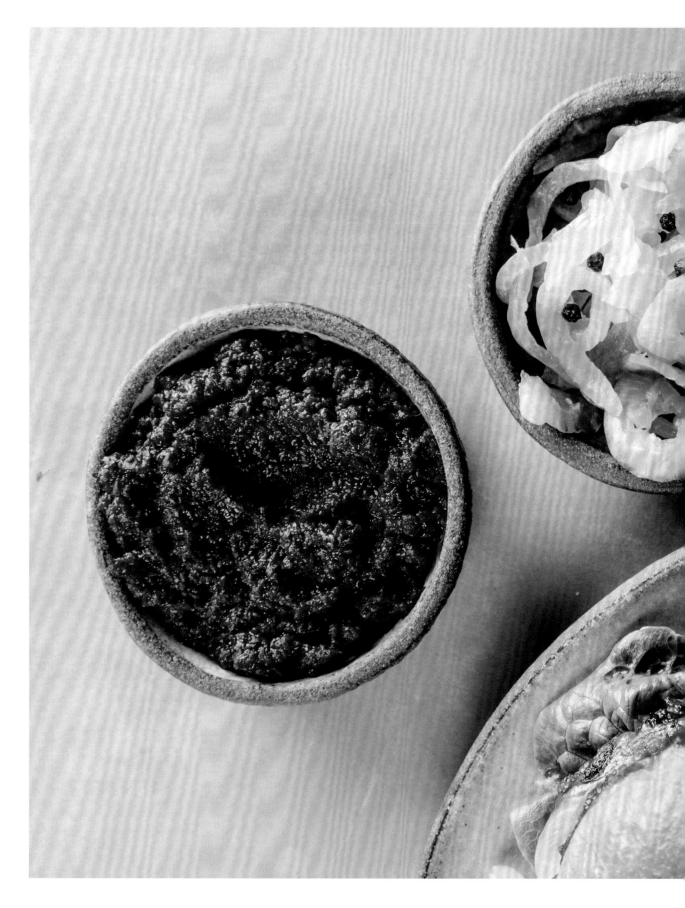

KETCHUP

2 tablespoons grapeseed oil or other neutral oil

120 grams coarsely chopped onion

30 grams coarsely chopped garlic (6 to 8 medium cloves)

650 grams canned whole or diced tomatoes (from one 28-ounce can), with their juices

120 grams tomato paste

2 teaspoons Chinese five-spice powder

2 teaspoons mustard powder

1 teaspoon freshly ground black pepper

1 teaspoon ground ginger

½ to 1 teaspoon ground chipotle chile powder

15 grams coarse unrefined sea salt

50 milliliters natural brine from Basic Kraut (page 92) or 50 grams Basic Kraut

EQUIPMENT

Kitchen scale

Food processor or blender

1-quart or 1-liter wide-mouth glass jar

Canning funnel (optional)

Parchment paper or cheesecloth cut to the diameter of the jar

Fermentation lid

It may surprise you to learn that the word *ketchup* comes from the Hokkien Chinese word *kê-tsiap*, which means "fermented fish sauce." The English, who likely encountered *kê-tsiap* in Southeast Asia, tried to replicate it with a variety of ingredients, like mushrooms, walnuts, oysters, and anchovies. The first recipe with tomatoes appeared in 1812, and in 1876, Henry J. Heinz introduced Americans to the tomato ketchup we know and love today. A whopping 97 percent of households report having a bottle of ketchup in their refrigerator.

Full disclosure: We are in the 3 percent who apparently did not get the ketchup-loving gene. We both find it too sweet, preferring mayonnaise with our fries, which completely grosses out most of our American friends. So why on Earth did we include a recipe for ketchup in this book? Both of us were absolutely fascinated by ketchup's fermented origins. We thought about trying to make the English mushroom ketchup that Jane Austen is purported to have loved, but then realized that the recipe would be too similar to our Mushroom Umami Sauce (page 232). But we were determined to come up with a more complex counterpart to an otherwise cloyingly sweet sauce (sorry, ketchup lovers!), so we set to work and eventually developed this recipe. Our concoction not only passes muster with lovers and nonlovers of Heinz, but it has become the most frequently requested recipe we make.

If you find that the ketchup isn't sweet enough post-fermentation, you can stir in a little honey or the sweetener of your choice. While this added sugar will help to balance the flavor of the ketchup, it will also be giving the microbes a fresh food supply, resulting in continued fermentation, and if it is in a sealed container, it can also cause carbonation to build up. For this reason, it is best to add the additional sweetener to the ketchup right before serving.

1. Wash and sanitize all your fermentation equipment and set aside to air-dry.

2. In a small skillet, warm the grapeseed oil over medium heat. Add the onion and cook, stirring, until translucent. Add the garlic and cook for another minute. Transfer the mixture to the food processor. Add the tomatoes with their juices, tomato paste, five-spice powder, mustard powder, pepper, ginger, chipotle, salt, and kraut brine and process into a smooth paste.

3. Transfer the ketchup to the jar (a canning funnel is useful here and helps to minimize spillage), making sure there are no air pockets and leaving 1 inch of headspace. Place the parchment paper or cheesecloth in the jar over the ketchup (the ketchup should be completely covered).

4. Ferment the ketchup in a cool place away from direct sunlight (4 days at 64°F is ideal—see the chart at right). Taste the ketchup after 3 days to determine if the flavor and sourness are to your liking. If it's not sour enough, reseal the jar and let the ketchup ferment for another day or two, then taste again.

5. When the flavor of the ketchup is sour to your liking, replace the fermentation lid with a regular lid and transfer the ketchup to the refrigerator. Let the flavors continue to develop for 2 to 3 days before using the ketchup. It will keep for 3 to 6 months. The less often you open the jar, the longer the ketchup will keep, so if you think you'll take your time getting through it, you may want to transfer the ketchup into two 1-pint or ½-liter jars.

Fermentation Temperature & Time

Above 68°F
Ferment 3 days or less

65° to 68°F
Ferment 3 to 4 days

Ideal: 64°F
Ferment 4 days

60° to 63°F
Ferment 4 to 5 days

Below 60°F
Ferment 5 days or more

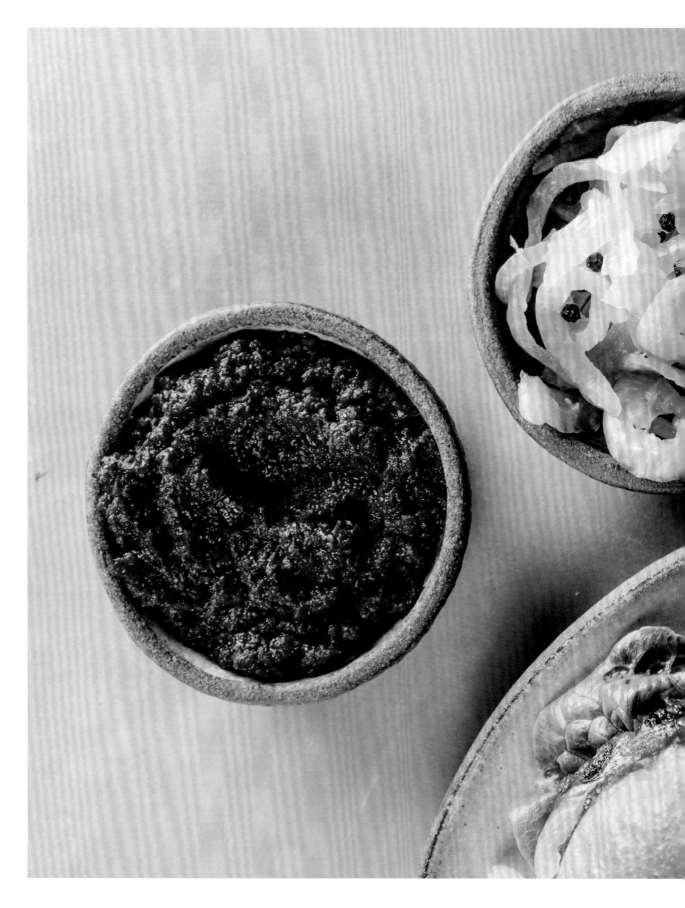

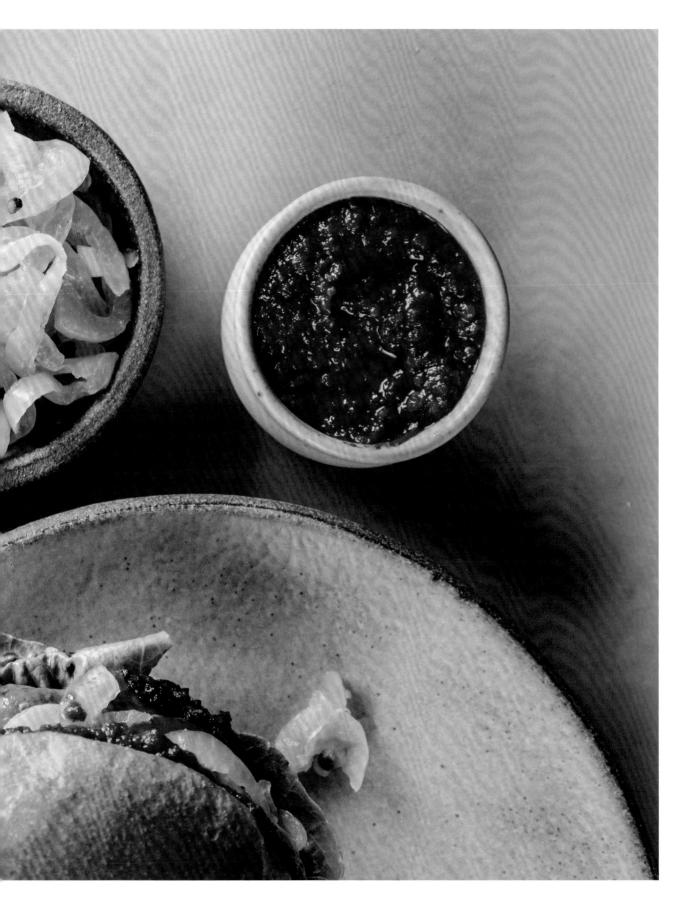

BEET-HORSERADISH MUSTARD

MAKES 1 QUART

400 grams shredded
peeled beets

400 grams yellow mustard seeds

20 grams coarse unrefined
sea salt

50 milliliters natural brine
from Basic Kraut (page 92)
or 50 grams Basic Kraut

100 grams Preserved
Horseradish Puree (page 176)
or store-bought prepared
horseradish

Honey, as needed (optional)

EQUIPMENT

Kitchen scale

Latex gloves

1-quart or 1-liter wide-mouth
glass jar

Canning funnel (optional)

Kraut tamper (optional)

Parchment paper or cheesecloth
cut to the diameter of the jar

Fermentation lid

Food processor or blender

Beet horseradish is a classic condiment used to add pep to gefilte fish during Passover and to cut the richness of ham in Easter meals. We love the way the two ingredients play off each other and thought they might also play nicely with mustard. The combination worked so well that it's now the only mustard we use.

1. Wash and sanitize all your fermentation equipment, including a medium bowl, knife, and cutting board, and set aside to air-dry.

2. In the medium bowl, combine the beets, mustard seeds, salt, and kraut brine. With gloved hands, massage, squeeze, and mix the beets until they begin to release liquid, about 5 minutes. When you can grab a handful of beets and squeeze the liquid out of it easily, it's ready to go.

3. Transfer the beets to the jar along with any liquid (a canning funnel is useful here and helps to minimize spillage). As you add the beets, tamp down with your fist or a kraut tamper to force out any air pockets. Continue until the jar is almost full, leaving 1 inch of headspace. Place the parchment paper or cheesecloth in the jar over the beets (the beets should be completely covered).

4. Seal the jar with the fermentation lid. Place the sealed jar in a bowl to catch any liquid displaced through the airlock during fermentation. Ferment the beet mustard in a cool place away from direct sunlight (3 weeks at 64°F is ideal—see the chart on page 160). Taste the beet mustard after 2 weeks. If it's not sour enough, reseal the jar and let it ferment for another week, then taste again.

5. When the beet mustard is sour to your liking, transfer it to a food processor or blender, add the horseradish puree, and process until the mixture is smooth. Open the processor, being careful not to inhale the fumes, and scrape down the sides of the processor bowl with a spatula. Process again until well blended and very smooth.

6. Taste the beet-horseradish mustard—if it's too bitter, add a small amount honey in 1-tablespoon increments until the desired flavor is achieved. (Honey is a food source for the bacteria, which can result in a slight effervescence so it's best to add the honey right before you serve the condiment or open the jar periodically to allow the gas to escape.) Replace the fermentation lid with a regular lid, seal, and store in the refrigerator for up to 10 months.

BLACK PEPPER ONIONS

MAKES 1 QUART

900 grams sliced onions
(¼-inch-thick slices)

20 grams coarse unrefined
sea salt

10 grams whole black
peppercorns

50 milliliters natural brine
from Basic Kraut (page 92)
or 50 grams Basic Kraut

EQUIPMENT

Kitchen scale

Latex gloves

1-quart or 1-liter wide-mouth
glass jar

Canning funnel (optional)

Kraut tamper (optional)

Weight

Fermentation lid

This ferment is so simple to make it will soon be a mainstay in your fridge. Any time you need onion for a recipe, you can pull a little out of the jar without the hassle of having to tearfully prep a raw one. These deliciously tangy onions also make a great addition to sandwiches and burgers, and are an excellent topper for hot dogs. Onions can sometimes get a little slimy during fermentation, but don't fret: this is likely dextran (see page 83), a naturally occurring sugar. Let the onions ferment for another week, and the slimy texture will break down and no longer be an issue.

A word of caution: While they're fermenting, the onions will make your whole house smell like a burger joint, so you may want to ferment them in someplace like the garage. And if you're worried about your hands smelling like onions, wear gloves while you prep the ferment.

1. Wash and sanitize all your fermentation equipment, including a medium bowl, knife, and cutting board, and set aside to air-dry.

2. In the medium bowl, combine the onions, salt, peppercorns, and kraut brine. With gloved hands, massage, squeeze, and mix the onions until they begin to release liquid, about 2 minutes. When you can grab a handful of onions and squeeze the liquid out of it easily, it's ready to go.

3. Transfer the onions to the jar along with any liquid (a canning funnel is useful here). As you add the onions, tamp them down with your fist or a kraut tamper to submerge the solids under the brine and force out any air pockets. Continue until the jar is almost full, leaving 1 to 2 inches of headspace.

4. Place the weight in the jar on top of the onions and press down until the onions are completely submerged in the brine. Seal the jar with the fermentation lid. Place the sealed jar in a bowl to catch any liquid displaced through the airlock during fermentation.

5. Ferment the onions in a cool place away from direct sunlight (3 weeks at 64°F is ideal—see the chart on page 160). Taste the onions after 2 weeks to determine if the flavor and sourness are to your liking. If they're not sour enough, reseal the jar and let them ferment for another week, then taste again. When the onions are sour to your liking, replace the fermentation lid with a regular lid, seal, and store in the refrigerator for up to 10 months.

300 grams peeled fresh
horseradish root

25 milliliters fresh lemon juice
(from about 1 lemon)

10 grams coarse unrefined
sea salt

140 milliliters natural brine from
Basic Kraut (page 92)

EQUIPMENT

Kitchen scale

Goggles

Surgical mask

Food processor with shredding
disk and chopping blade

1-pint or ½-liter wide-mouth
glass jar with lid

Canning funnel (optional)

Parchment paper or cheesecloth
cut to the diameter of the jar

PRESERVED HORSERADISH PUREE

We think horseradish is an underutilized aromatic in American cooking.
Not only does its pungency complement fatty meats and a number of other
foods, but the list of its health benefits is truly impressive. Though it's an
excellent expectorant, its powerful antimicrobial properties have been most
prized through the ages. These compounds are thought to protect against
listeria, *E. coli*, *Staphylococcus aureus*, and other foodborne bacteria, and
may explain why horseradish has been served alongside meat and fish since
the Middle Ages. Horseradish is also considered to be cancer-protective.

Horseradish is traditionally prepared with vinegar to preserve its sharp,
pungent flavor, but it turns out that kraut brine is an excellent stand-in.
The flavor is milder and less bracing, and we are happy to report that even
though horseradish is antimicrobial, the live cultures in this puree survive
for several months. By making your own puree, you're not only adding
probiotics, but also eliminating a number of unpronounceable ingredients
that have been added to commercially prepared horseradish in recent
years. Simply process the horseradish and soak it in brine—no fermenting
necessary.

Depending on where you live, the fresh root is typically harvested in spring
and fall and kept in cold storage between harvests. The longer the root sits
in storage, the milder it gets. We typically make puree in early spring so
we can have a fresh jar for Easter and for the Passover table, then make it
again in the fall time so we have enough to get through the winter.

Caution: You *must* process the fresh horseradish root outside, or in a very
well-ventilated room. When the root is cut, the compound allyl isothiocya-
nate is released into the air and can irritate the mucous membranes in your
eyes and nose and even cause nausea. Eye protection is mandatory—swim
goggles or a dive mask work well—and wearing a surgical mask to protect
your sinuses is recommended, especially if you're processing the horseradish indoors. Leave your goggles and mask on during cleanup. Make
sure that pets and children are sequestered from the area before you start.
With the proper precautions, this process is safe and quick, and we think
the final result is well worth the extra effort.

1. Wash and sanitize all your fermentation equipment, including a medium bowl, knife, and cutting board, and set aside to air-dry.

2. Set up your food processor in a well-ventilated room or, even better, outside. Fit the processor with the shredding disk and have the chopping blade nearby. Put on the goggles and mask and make sure they're secure.

3. Cut the peeled horseradish root into chunks just small enough to fit into the food processor chute. Using the food processor, shred all the horseradish. Working quickly, transfer the shredded horseradish to the medium bowl. Without rinsing the food processor bowl, put the chopping blade in place and return the shredded horseradish to the processor bowl. Add the lemon juice and salt and process until the horseradish is pureed. Transfer the puree back to the bowl and gently stir the kraut brine into the mixture.

4. Transfer the horseradish puree to the jar, along with any liquid (a canning funnel is useful here and helps to minimize spillage), tamping down the mixture as you go to make sure there are no air pockets and leaving 1 inch of headspace. Place the parchment paper or cheesecloth in the jar over the horseradish (the horseradish should be completely covered). Seal the jar with a regular lid. (It's now safe to remove the goggles and mask.) Store the horseradish puree in the refrigerator for up to 6 months.

Note: Use cool to warm water for washing down your equipment, as hot water can aerosolize the horseradish fumes and cause irritation.

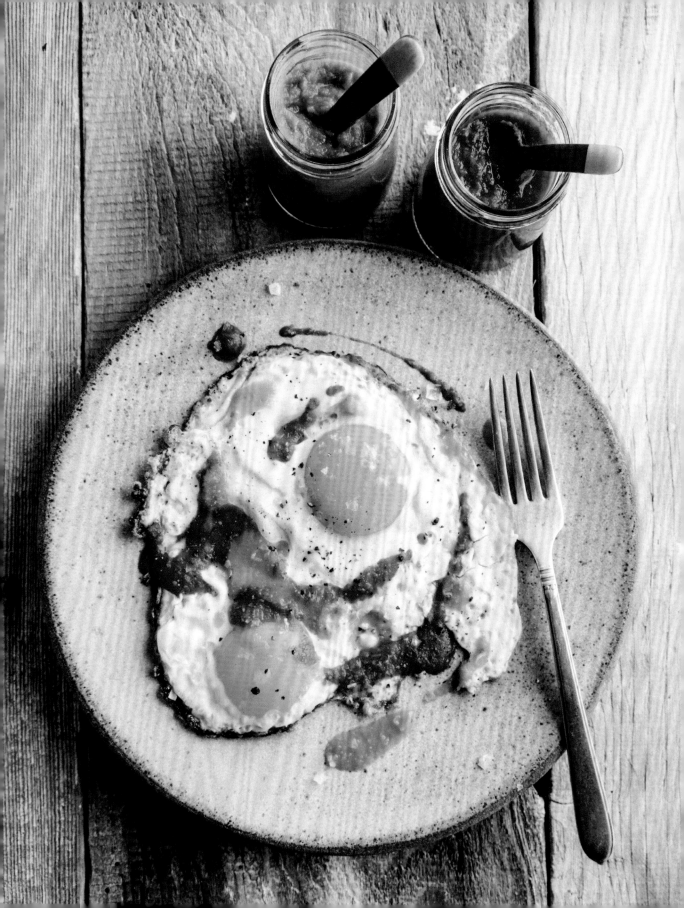

Pepper Mashes and Hot Sauces

Most hot sauces start their fiery lives in crocks or barrels as pepper mashes. Chopped, salted, and left to stew in their own juices for months or, in some cases, years, fermented peppers were likely the first pickled peppers that Peter perfected. The modern hot sauces found on grocery store shelves and restaurant tables are generally pasteurized and acidified with vinegar, and yet the base of most these sauces, a long-fermented/aged pepper mash, is quite another thing entirely. The complex and nuanced umami flavor that develops over the course of a long fermentation period is reason enough to ferment your peppers. There is also an added health bonus: probiotic bacteria, enzymes, and vitamin C, normally lost in pasteurization, are all preserved through the fermentation process. Every recipe in this section can simply be enjoyed as a pepper mash, an underutilized and delicious condiment that can be used on any dish to add a touch of spice, or you can choose to transform the pepper mashes into hot sauces.

It seems that just about every culture around the world makes a spicy condiment, and deciding which ones to include in this book came down to a desire to provide you with a diverse sampling, from simple to more complex. In truth, we can't think of a style of hot sauce that wouldn't thrive in a crock (or jar). If you don't see your favorite type here, find a recipe for a nonfermented version and follow our basic instructions to give it a shot. You might even find that your fermented version is better—it will certainly be healthier!

FERMENTER'S NOTES

Produce: When it comes to choosing peppers, the varieties are nearly as endless as their characteristics. You can make single-pepper mashes and enjoy their individual personalities, or you can blend them with other fermented peppers post-fermentation to achieve just the right balance of flavors. Growing conditions can significantly impact the flavor and heat of a pepper, which was an ongoing challenge for us in the early days of buying jalapeños for our Smoked Jalapeño Kraut. Early in the season, peppers can taste vegetal and have very little heat, but as the season progresses, the warmth of the sun increases their sweetness and heat. For this reason, you'll want to taste your peppers before you start prepping them, keeping in mind that the pith and seeds are where most of the heat resides and the bottom tip is the mildest part of the pepper.

When it comes to heat, some peppers make your lips tingle, others spark the tip of your tongue, and many, like jalapeños, are slow to come on but long to finish. You can easily find charts online that will help you determine the level of heat for different varieties of peppers, measured in Scoville units (a measure of their relative heat), but remember that these units are estimates at best and a pepper's heat can fluctuate based on a multitude of factors.

Finally, working with peppers in large batches can be challenging, so please read the safety guidelines below before starting.

Brine: The water content of peppers can vary due to season, growing practices, and variety. If your peppers do not initially produce enough liquid to fully submerge the mash, you can make extra brine to top it off—in most cases, 100 grams of brine should be enough. Simply dissolve 3 grams salt in 97 milliliters filtered water and fill the jar with the brine, leaving 2 inches of headspace. This brine can also be used if you lose some of the brine through the airlock or lid during the fermentation process. If this happens, open the jar, add the replacement bring, again leaving 2 inches of headspace, and reseal (leave the jar open only as long as it takes to add the brine, to avoid introducing unwanted yeasts and molds). During the first one to two weeks, gas (CO_2) is produced, which can cause the brine to be expelled through the airlock, potentially dropping the brine level below the mash. If you add replacement brine too soon, it will just be expelled by the gases too, so wait until the end of this first phase before adding more brine. The exposed mash is protected by a layer of CO_2 during this phase and generally will not deteriorate. You'll know this phase is complete when the brine stops bubbling. (Liquid loss will slow after the first two weeks as the fermentation process slows).

Safety: Capsaicin, one of the primary active components in chile peppers, is the compound responsible for the heat that those of us who love spicy foods have come to enjoy. But capsaicin is an irritant and will cause a burning sensation on any skin tissue it comes in contact with, and that heat you love in your food is not very pleasant when it involves other parts of you body. But don't worry—just take the proper precautions, and soon you'll be enjoying the best hot sauces you've ever tasted.

First, always wear gloves when you are handling peppers.

When blending or processing peppers, be careful not to inhale the fumes that are the result of the peppers releasing their capsaicin into the air. Breathing in aerosolized capsaicin will make you cough and choke, and can also irritate your eyes.

Do *not* touch your eyes, or any other sensitive areas, after handling peppers, and thoroughly wash your hands before touching any other part of your body.

Last, when cleaning your food processor, bowls, or other tools after a pepper-processing session, always use cold water to do the majority of the washing, since hot water can aerosolize the capsaicin.

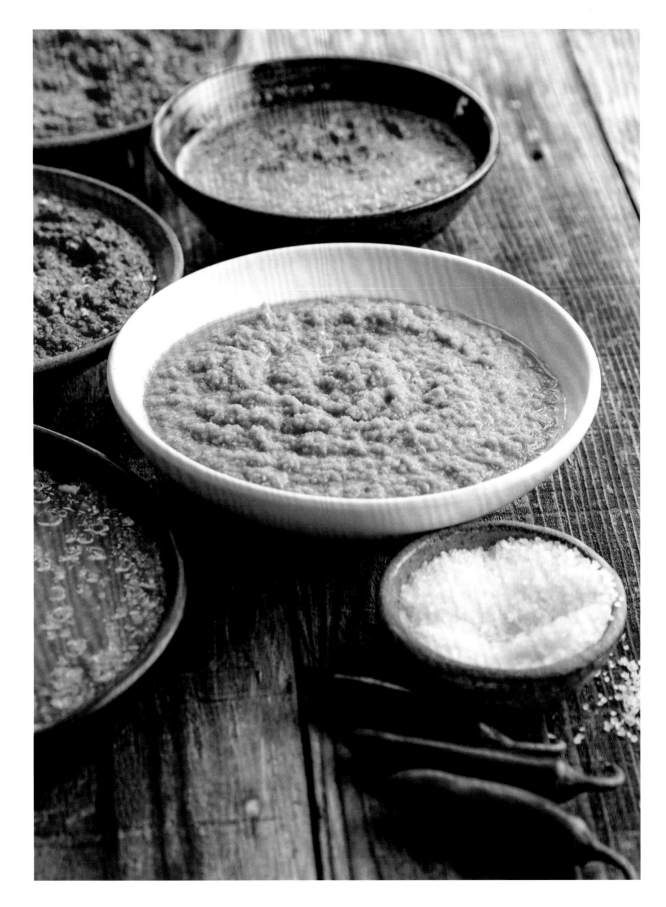

BASIC PEPPER MASH OR HOT SAUCE

MAKES 1 QUART

970 grams coarsely chopped green or red jalapeños, including seeds

30 grams coarse unrefined sea salt

EQUIPMENT

Kitchen scale

Latex gloves

Food processor or blender

1-quart or 1-liter wide-mouth glass jar

Canning funnel (optional)

Parchment paper or cheesecloth cut to the diameter of the jar

Fermentation lid

Smaller bottles or jars with lids, for storage

This basic pepper mash is as simple as it gets—salt and fresh peppers pureed into a spicy mash—but the resulting flavor is quite complex and anything but basic. It's truly amazing that two ingredients can be transformed into such a flavorful condiment with nothing more than salt and the transformative power of lactic acid bacteria. Within this recipe framework of 97 percent peppers to 3 percent salt, you can substitute a wide variety of pepper varieties as well as other additions such as herbs, spices, fruits, and vegetables, as you will see in our many variations that follow, to make your own unique pepper mashes and hot sauces. While it's fun and novel to play with making flavored pepper mashes, we keep coming back to this basic recipe as our go-to for making pepper mashes, substituting whatever pepper variety is inspiring us or looking particularly enticing throughout the season.

1. Wash and sanitize all your fermentation equipment, including a knife and cutting board, and set aside to air-dry.

2. Put the peppers in the food processor or blender, add the salt, and process for 2 to 3 minutes, until the mash is smooth. (The larger pepper pieces will often float to the top of the mash in the food processor, so alternate running the motor and pulsing to be sure they're incorporated.) Open the processor, being careful not to inhale the pepper fumes, and scrape down the sides of the processor bowl with a spatula. Process for 1 to 2 minutes more, until the mash is quite liquid.

3. Transfer the pepper mash to the jar along with any liquid (a canning funnel is useful here and helps to minimize spillage), pushing it down with a spatula or wooden spoon to remove any air pockets and leaving 1 inch of headspace. Place the parchment paper or cheesecloth in the jar over the mash (the mash should be completely covered).

4. Seal the jar with the fermentation lid. Place the sealed jar on a plate or in a bowl to catch any liquid displaced through the airlock during fermentation.

5. Ferment the pepper mash in a cool place away from direct sunlight for 1 to 3 months, depending on the

fermentation temperature (2 months at 64°F is ideal—see the chart at right). Keep an eye on the mash through the first 2 weeks—if it loses enough liquid during the first phase of fermentation that the top layer is exposed, top it off with brine (see Fermenter's Notes, page 181). Also, keep an eye on the airlock to make sure it never runs dry, cleaning it and refilling with fresh water as needed. Taste the pepper mash after 1 month to determine if the flavor is to your liking. If it's not, reseal the jar and leave to ferment for another month, then taste again. (We've found that 2 months is usually sufficient, but, to a certain degree, pepper mash just keeps getting better with age. The best pepper mash we ever made was fermented for over a year!)

6. When the pepper mash is to your liking, replace the fermentation lid with a regular lid, seal, and store in the refrigerator for up to 1 year, though it will likely last much longer.

7. If you would like to turn the mash into hot sauce, transfer it to a blender or food processor and puree until smooth. Strain the puree through a fine-mesh sieve into a bowl, pressing down on the solids with a wooden spoon to extract as much liquid as possible (reserve the spent solids to make a pepper seasoning, if you like—see Note). Transfer the liquid hot sauce into bottles or jars, seal, and store in the refrigerator for up to 1 year.

Note: Don't throw away the solids in the strainer! You can turn the spent mash into a delicious probiotic pepper seasoning. Simply spread the mash over dehydrator sheets in a thin layer and dehydrate at 110°F for 4 to 6 hours (alternatively, spread it over a baking sheet and dry it in the sun, until the liquid has evaporated). Transfer the dried pepper mash to a spice grinder or a mortar and pestle and grind it into a powder. Transfer the ground pepper into small jars and store in a cool, dark place with your other spices for up to 1 year.

Fermentation Temperature & Time

Above 68°F
Ferment 1 month or less

65° to 68°F
Ferment 1 to 2 months

Ideal: 64°F
Ferment 2 months

60° to 63°F
Ferment 2 to 3 months

Below 60°F
Ferment 3 months or more

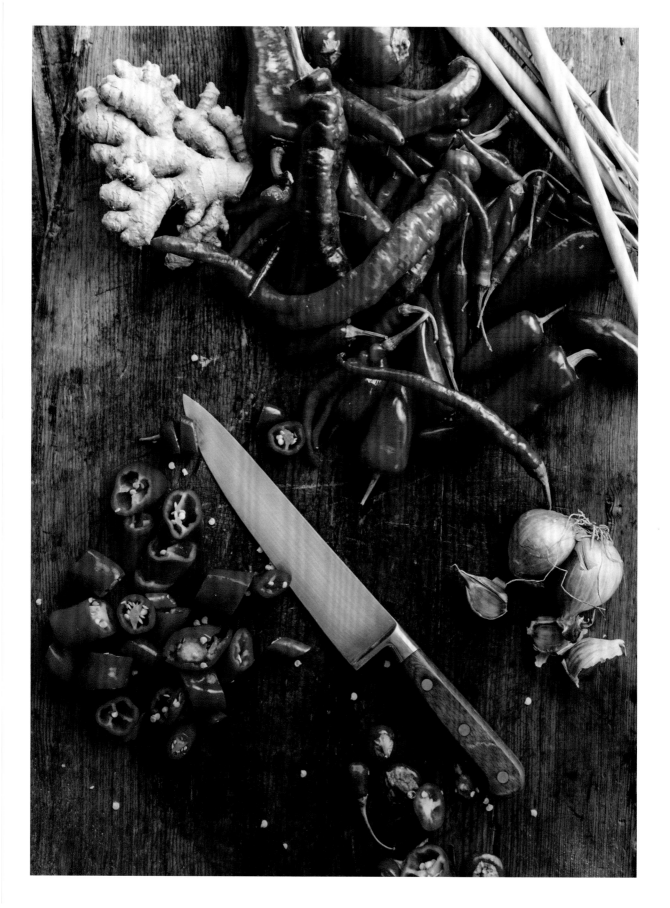

SAMBAL BALI-CALI

MAKES 1 QUART

820 grams coarsely chopped hot red peppers (Thai, serrano, or red jalapeño), including seeds

50 grams coarsely chopped shallots

30 grams coarsely chopped garlic

30 grams coarsely chopped peeled fresh ginger

20 grams coarsely chopped lemongrass (about 2 stalks)

20 grams tamarind paste

30 grams coarse unrefined sea salt

EQUIPMENT

Kitchen scale

Latex gloves

Food processor or blender

1-quart or 1-liter wide-mouth glass jar

Canning funnel (optional)

Parchment paper or cheesecloth cut to the diameter of the jar

Fermentation lid

Never heard of Sambal Bali-Cali? You're not alone. There are so many sambals out there, we decided to throw one more in the mix. You might be familiar with sambal oelek, a basic but delicious Southeast Asian chile sauce that's readily available in most grocery stores. Our sambal is based on a Balinese version called *sambal matah*. We changed a couple of ingredients and took liberties with the quantities—and depending on your tolerance for heat, you might be happy we did. The original recipe calls for birds-eye chiles, which will burn your tongue off if you're not careful. After four generations in California, we had to slip a little Mexican tamarind paste in, hence the Cali part. It adds a little sweet and sour, bringing balance and a welcome calm to the sauce. We took that revised mix, fermented it, and voilà—Sambal Bali-Cali was born.

Fantastic in stir-fries and marinades, Sambal Bali-Cali really can be used just about anywhere you want a little bright heat. Remember, though, that even with milder peppers, a little goes a long way.

1. Wash and sanitize all your fermentation equipment, including a knife and cutting board, and set aside to air-dry.

2. Put the peppers in the food processor or blender; add the shallots, garlic, ginger, lemongrass, tamarind paste, and salt; and process for 2 to 3 minutes, until the mash is smooth. (The larger pepper pieces will often float to the top of the mash in the food processor, so alternate running the motor and pulsing to be sure they're incorporated.) Open the processor, being careful not to inhale the pepper fumes, and scrape down the sides of the processor bowl with a spatula. Process for 1 to 2 minutes more, until the mash is quite liquid.

3. Transfer the pepper mash to the jar along with any liquid (a canning funnel is useful here and helps to minimize spillage), pushing it down with a spatula or wooden spoon to remove any air pockets and leaving 1 inch of headspace. Place the parchment paper or cheesecloth in the jar over the mash (the mash should be completely covered).

4. Seal the jar with the fermentation lid. Place the sealed jar on a plate or in a bowl to catch any liquid displaced through the airlock during fermentation.

CONTINUED ›

5. Ferment the pepper mash in a cool place away from direct sunlight (2 months at 64°F is ideal—see the chart on page 185). Keep an eye on the mash through the first 2 weeks— if it loses enough liquid during the first phase of fermentation that the top layer is exposed, top it off with brine (see Fermenter's Notes, page 181). Also, keep an eye on the airlock to make sure it never runs dry, cleaning it and refilling with fresh water as needed. Taste the pepper mash after 1 month to determine if the flavor is to your liking. If it's not, reseal the jar and leave to ferment for another month, then taste again. When the pepper mash is to your liking, replace the fermentation lid with a regular lid, seal, and store in the refrigerator for up to 1 year, though it will likely last much longer.

6. To turn the mash into hot sauce, see step 7 on page 185.

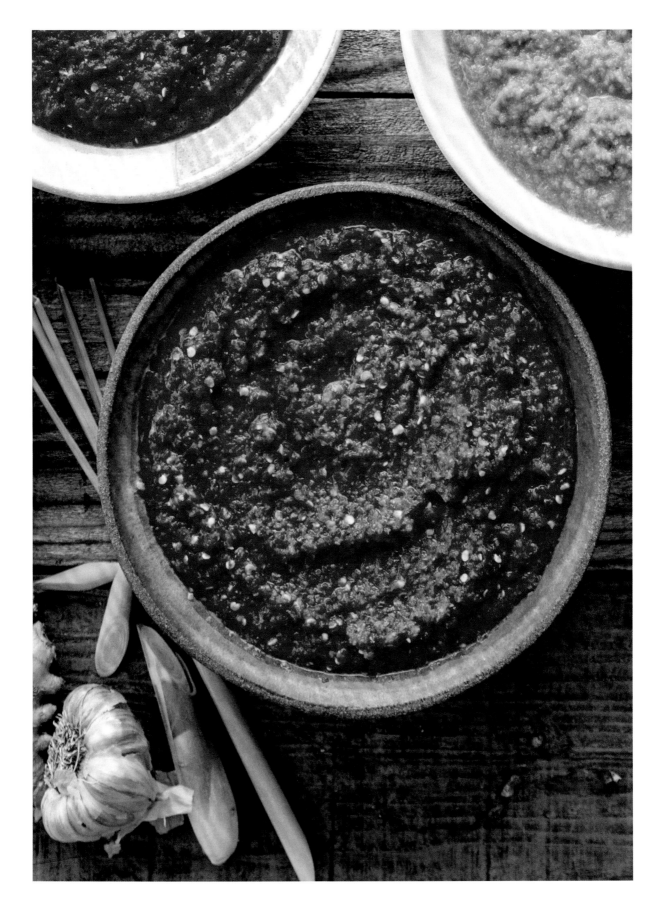

JAMAICAN-STYLE HOT SAUCE

450 grams coarsely chopped
red jalapeño peppers,
including seeds

300 grams fresh or canned
diced red tomatoes, drained

100 grams coarsely chopped
white or yellow onion

50 grams chopped fresh mango

30 grams coarsely chopped
peeled fresh ginger

20 grams raisins

2 teaspoons orange zest

1 teaspoon minced fresh thyme

1 teaspoon freshly ground
black pepper

½ teaspoon ground cloves

30 grams coarse unrefined
sea salt

EQUIPMENT

Kitchen scale

Latex gloves

Food processor or blender

1-quart or 1-liter wide-mouth
glass jar

Canning funnel (optional)

Parchment paper or cheesecloth
cut to the diameter of the jar

Fermentation lid

Smaller bottles or jars with lids,
for storage

We developed this recipe to mimic the flavors and style of Pickapeppa sauce, a popular Jamaican brand. Commonly poured over cream cheese and used as a spread, this unique sauce has tropical notes from the mango and ginger, balanced by the sweetness of tomatoes and raisins, and the aromatic spices. We used the classic and easily procured jalapeño, but you can substitute any hot pepper you like.

1. Wash and sanitize all your fermentation equipment, including a knife and cutting board, and set aside to air-dry.

2. Put the peppers in the food processor or blender; add the tomatoes, onion, mango, ginger, raisins, orange zest; thyme, black pepper, cloves, and salt, and process for 2 to 3 minutes, until the mash is smooth. (The larger pepper pieces will often float to the top of the mash in the food processor, so alternate running the motor and pulsing to be sure they're incorporated.) Open the processor, being careful not to inhale the pepper fumes, and scrape down the sides of the processor bowl with a spatula. Process for 1 to 2 minutes more, until the mash is quite liquid.

3. Transfer the pepper mash to the jar along with any liquid (a canning funnel is useful here), pushing it down with a spatula or wooden spoon to remove any air pockets and leaving 1 inch of headspace. Place the parchment paper or cheesecloth in the jar over the mash (the mash should be completely covered). Seal the jar with the fermentation lid. Place the sealed jar on a plate or in a bowl to catch any liquid displaced through the airlock during fermentation.

4. Ferment the pepper mash in a cool place away from direct sunlight (2 months at 64°F is ideal—see the chart on page 185). Keep an eye on the mash through the first 2 weeks— if it loses enough liquid during the first phase of fermentation that the top layer is exposed, top it off with brine (see Fermenter's Notes, page 181). Also, keep an eye on the airlock to make sure it never runs dry, cleaning it and refilling with fresh water as needed. Taste the pepper mash after 1 month to determine if the flavor is to your liking. If it's not, reseal the jar and leave to ferment for another month, then taste again. When the pepper mash is to your liking, transfer it to a blender and puree into a thick sauce. Transfer the sauce into bottles or jars, seal, and store in the refrigerator for at least 1 year, though it will likely last much longer.

EROS PISTA

MAKES 1 QUART

820 grams coarsely chopped
red bell peppers

150 grams Hungarian
hot paprika

30 grams coarse unrefined
sea salt

EQUIPMENT

Kitchen scale

Food processor or blender

1-quart or 1-liter wide-mouth
glass jar

Canning funnel (optional)

Parchment paper or cheesecloth
cut to the diameter of the jar

Fermentation lid

Eros pista is a classic Hungarian pepper paste, often sold in tubes and typically used in dishes such as chicken paprikash, goulash, and ragout. Traditionally, this paste is fermented with fresh hot paprika peppers and salt, but because we were not able find these peppers, we came up with what we think is a pretty darned good alternative. Hungarian hot paprika is available online and in specialty stores. Make sure you get the spicy one!

1. Wash and sanitize all your fermentation equipment, including a knife and cutting board, and set aside to air-dry.

2. Put the bell peppers in your food processor or blender, add the paprika and salt, and process for 2 to 3 minutes, until the mash is smooth. (The larger pepper pieces will often float to the top of the mash in the food processor, so alternate running the motor and pulsing to be sure they're incorporated.) Open the processor and scrape down the sides of the processor bowl with a spatula. Process for 1 to 2 minutes more, until the mash is quite liquid.

3. Transfer the pepper mash to the jar along with any liquid (a canning funnel is useful here and helps to minimize spillage), pushing it down with a spatula or wooden spoon to remove any air pockets and leaving 1 inch of headspace. Place the parchment paper or cheesecloth in the jar over the mash (the mash should be completely covered). Seal the jar with the fermentation lid. Place the sealed jar in a bowl to catch any liquid displaced through the airlock during fermentation.

4. Ferment the pepper mash in a cool place away from direct sunlight (2 months at 64°F is ideal—see the chart on page 185). Keep an eye on the mash through the first 2 weeks—if it loses enough liquid during the first phase of fermentation that the top layer is exposed, top it off with brine (see Fermenter's Notes, page 181). Also, keep an eye on the airlock to make sure it never runs dry, cleaning it and refilling with fresh water as needed. Taste the pepper mash after 1 month to determine if the flavor is to your liking. If it's not, reseal the jar and leave to ferment for another month, then taste again. When the pepper mash is to your liking, replace the fermentation lid with a regular lid, seal, and store in the refrigerator for up to 1 year, though it will likely last much longer.

5. To turn the mash into hot sauce, see step 7 on page 185.

HARISSA

500 milliliters filtered water

100 grams dried red chiles
(see Note)

10 grams cumin seeds

10 grams caraway seeds

10 grams coriander seeds

250 grams coarsely chopped
red bell pepper

250 grams coarsely chopped
serrano pepper

40 grams coarsely
chopped garlic

30 grams coarse unrefined
sea salt

EQUIPMENT

Kitchen scale

Latex gloves

Spice grinder or mortar
and pestle

Food processor or blender

1-quart or 1-liter wide-mouth
glass jar

Canning funnel (optional)

Parchment paper or cheesecloth
cut to the diameter of the jar

Fermentation lid

Harissa is one the first pepper sauces we ever made, and it continues to be a favorite. Traditionally preserved in oil rather than fermented, this smoky North African chile sauce is widely used in Tunisian and, more recently, Moroccan cuisine. We think fermenting the chiles creates an umami profile that adds depth to this already flavorful sauce.

If you're sensitive to heat, kick up the bell peppers and minimize the serranos. The dried chiles are quite mild—and whatever you do, don't throw out their soaking liquid. The flavor is incredible. Not only will you need it to get the consistency of the paste right, but you can add it to soups and sauces, and might even be tempted to drink it straight like we did when working on this recipe.

This sauce tends to be quite thick—more of a paste really, which makes it great for basting chicken, fish, and vegetables. Just go easy, it's pretty fiery.

1. Wash and sanitize all your fermentation equipment, including a large bowl, knife, and cutting board, and set aside to air-dry.

2. Put the water in a medium saucepan, cover, and bring to a boil. Remove from the heat and add the dried chiles. Cover and let soak for 20 minutes.

3. Toast the cumin, caraway, and coriander in a dry skillet over medium heat until they turn golden. Transfer to a small plate and let cool, then finely grind in a spice grinder or using a mortar and pestle.

4. Drain the chiles in a fine-mesh sieve set over the large bowl; reserve the soaking liquid. Transfer the rehydrated chiles and 250 milliliters of the soaking water to the food processor or blender. Add the ground cumin, caraway, and coriander, plus the bell pepper, serrano, garlic, and salt and process for 2 to 3 minutes, until the mixture forms a smooth paste. If the mixture is too thick and you are having trouble blending it, add more chile soaking liquid as needed, 100 milliliters at a time. (The larger pepper pieces will often float to the top of the mash in the food

processor, so alternate running the motor and pulsing to be sure they're incorporated.) Open the processor, being careful not to inhale the pepper fumes, and scrape down the sides of the processor bowl with a spatula. Process for 1 to 2 minutes more, until the mash is quite liquid.

5. Transfer the pepper mash to the jar along with any liquid (a canning funnel is useful here and helps to minimize spillage), pushing it down with a spatula or wooden spoon to remove any air pockets and leaving 1 inch of headspace. Place the parchment paper or cheesecloth in the jar over the mash (the mash should be completely covered). Seal the jar with the fermentation lid. Place the sealed jar on a plate or in a bowl to catch any liquid displaced through the airlock during fermentation.

6. Ferment the pepper mash in a cool place away from direct sunlight (2 months at 64°F is ideal—see the chart on page 185). Keep an eye on the mash through the first 2 weeks— if it loses enough liquid during the first phase of fermentation that the top layer is exposed, top it off with brine (see Fermenter's Notes, page 181). Also, keep an eye on the airlock to make sure it never runs dry, cleaning it and refilling with fresh water as needed. Taste the pepper mash after 1 month to determine if the flavor is to your liking. If it's not, reseal the jar and leave to ferment for another month, then taste again. When the pepper mash is to your liking, replace the fermentation lid with a regular lid, seal, and store in the refrigerator for up to 1 year, though it will likely last much longer.

7. To turn the mash into hot sauce, see step 7 on page 185.

Note: Unless you have access to a Moroccan or Tunisian store, it's unlikely you'll be able to find North African dried chiles—but don't worry. Many other dried chiles are readily available and just as delicious. We like a combination of New Mexico for their mellow heat, ancho for their depth, and a little chipotle for smokiness. We found all three in the Mexican section of a local grocer.

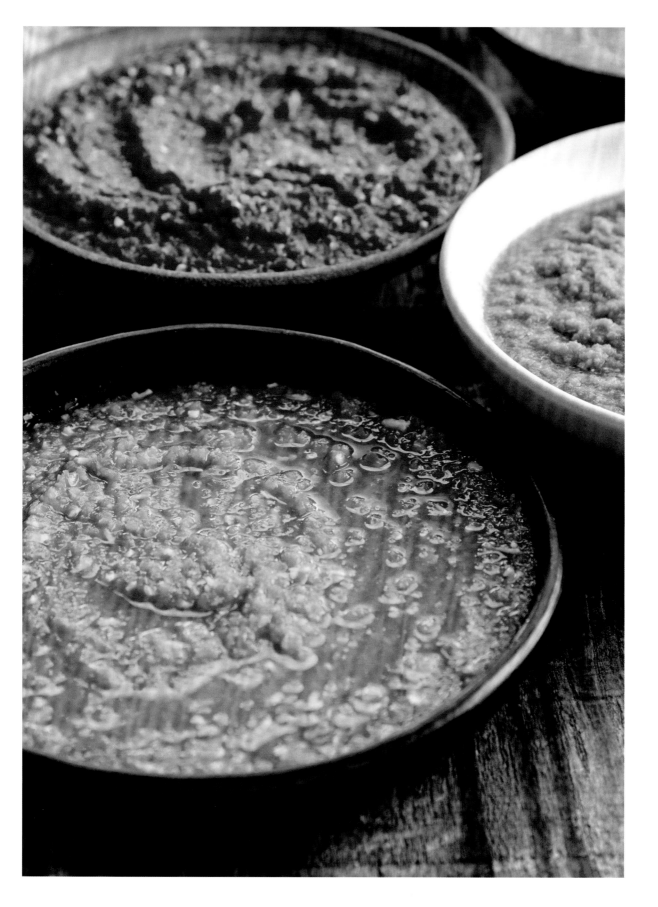

CARROT-COCONUT PEPPER MASH

MAKES 1 QUART

580 grams coarsely chopped orange or yellow bell peppers

100 grams coarsely chopped habanero peppers, including seeds

150 grams coarsely chopped carrots

70 grams coarsely chopped fresh or frozen mango

30 grams coarsely chopped peeled fresh ginger

10 grams unsweetened flaked or shredded coconut

1 teaspoon lime zest

25 milliliters lime juice (from about 1 lime)

30 grams coarse unrefined sea salt

EQUIPMENT

Kitchen scale

Latex gloves

Food processor or blender

1-quart or 1-liter wide-mouth glass jar

Canning funnel (optional)

Parchment paper or cheesecloth cut to the diameter of the jar

Fermentation lid

Using mostly bell peppers to balance the intense heat of the habanero makes this hot sauce approachable for those who don't want to blow their head off with spice (like Kathryn). My fellow spice addicts out there can increase the habanero and decrease the bell peppers proportionally without negatively affecting the integrity of the ferment. —Shane

1. Wash and sanitize all your fermentation equipment, including a knife and cutting board, and set aside to air-dry.

2. Put the peppers in the food processor or blender; add the carrots, mango, ginger, coconut, lime zest, lime juice, and salt; and process for 2 to 3 minutes, until the mash is smooth. (The larger pepper pieces will often float to the top of the mash in the food processor, so alternate running the motor and pulsing to be sure they're incorporated.) Open the processor, being careful not to inhale the pepper fumes, and scrape down the sides of the processor bowl with a spatula. Process for 1 to 2 minutes more, until the mash is quite liquid.

3. Transfer the pepper mash to the jar along with any liquid (a canning funnel is useful here and helps to minimize spillage), pushing it down with a spatula or wooden spoon to remove any air pockets and leaving 1 inch of headspace. Place the parchment paper or cheesecloth in the jar over the mash (the mash should be completely covered). Seal the jar with the fermentation lid. Place the sealed jar in a bowl to catch any liquid displaced through the airlock during fermentation.

4. Ferment the pepper mash in a cool place away from direct sunlight (2 months at 64°F is ideal—see the chart on page 185). Keep an eye on the mash through the first 2 weeks—if it loses enough liquid during the first phase of fermentation that the top layer is exposed, top it off with brine (see Fermenter's Notes, page 181). Also, keep an eye on the airlock to make sure it never runs dry, cleaning it and refilling with fresh water as needed. Taste the pepper mash after 1 month to determine if the flavor is to your liking. If it's not, reseal the jar and leave to ferment for another month, then taste again. When the pepper mash is to your liking, replace the fermentation lid with a regular lid, seal, and store in the refrigerator for up to 1 year, though it will likely last much longer.

5. To turn the mash into hot sauce, see step 7 on page 185.

BARBADOS-STYLE HOT SAUCE

MAKES 1 QUART

700 grams coarsely chopped orange bell peppers

100 grams coarsely chopped Scotch bonnet or habanero peppers, including seeds

80 grams coarsely chopped yellow onion

80 grams coarsely chopped peeled fresh turmeric

2 teaspoons yellow mustard powder

30 grams coarse unrefined sea salt

EQUIPMENT

Kitchen scale

Latex gloves

Food processor or blender

1-quart or 1-liter wide-mouth glass jar

Canning funnel (optional)

Parchment paper or cheesecloth cut to the diameter of the jar

Fermentation lid

Fine-mesh sieve

Smaller bottles or jars with lids, for storage

If you are a masochistic spice lover as I am, then this is the hot sauce for you! We have adapted this recipe from the traditional Bajan hot sauce of Barbados, where it is served with everything and is traditionally made with the very spicy Scotch bonnet peppers (80,000 to 400,000 Scoville units!). We couldn't find Scotch bonnet peppers at our local grocer, so we substituted habaneros, which are similar in taste and spice level. Using just the habaneros, the sauce was so hot that even my spice-loving palate could not handle the heat. To make it more palatable, we decided to substitute orange bell peppers for some of the habaneros, which not only cuts the heat but also cuts your prep time and adds more liquid to the sauce. The combination of turmeric and mustard makes this beautiful yellow pepper sauce both unique and pungently delicious.

For spice lovers, it can be a point of pride to eat pure fire. This is the hottest pepper recipe we have come across, so if you really want to blow your taste buds away, try it with all habaneros, or a higher ratio of habaneros to bell peppers. But don't say we didn't warn you! —Shane

1. Wash and sanitize all your fermentation equipment, including a knife and cutting board, and set aside to air-dry.

2. Put the peppers in the food processor or blender; add the onion, turmeric, mustard powder, and salt; and process for 2 to 3 minutes, until the mash is smooth. (The larger pepper pieces will often float to the top of the mash in the food processor, so alternate running the motor and pulsing to be sure they're incorporated.) Open the processor, being careful not to inhale the pepper fumes, and scrape down the sides of the processor bowl with a spatula. Process for

1 to 2 minutes more, until the mash is quite liquid.

3. Transfer the pepper mash to the jar along with any liquid (a canning funnel is useful here and helps to minimize spillage), pushing it down with a spatula or wooden spoon to remove any air pockets and leaving 1 inch of headspace. Place the parchment paper or cheesecloth in the jar over the mash (the mash should be completely covered).

4. Seal the jar with the fermentation lid. Place the sealed jar on a plate or in a bowl to catch any liquid displaced through the airlock during fermentation.

5. Ferment the pepper mash in a cool place away from direct sunlight (2 months at 64°F is ideal—see the chart on page 185). Keep an eye on the mash through the first 2 weeks—if it loses enough liquid during the first phase of fermentation that the top layer is exposed, top it off with brine (see Fermenter's Notes, page 181). Also, keep an eye on the airlock to make sure it never runs dry, cleaning it and refilling with fresh water as needed. Taste the pepper mash after 1 month to determine if the flavor is to your liking. If it's not, reseal the jar and leave to ferment for another month, then taste again. When the pepper mash is to your liking, strain it through a fine-mesh sieve into a bowl, pressing down on the solids with a wooden spoon to extract as much liquid as possible (reserve the spent solids to make a pepper seasoning, if you like—see Note, page 185). Transfer the liquid hot sauce into smaller bottles or jars, seal, and store in the refrigerator. It will keep for at least 10 months.

CALIFORNIA-STYLE HOT SAUCE

2 teaspoons coriander seeds

2 teaspoons cumin seeds

750 grams coarsely chopped green jalapeños, including seeds

120 milliliters filtered water

30 grams ground chipotle chile powder or any red chile powder

30 grams chopped fresh garlic

20 grams dried garlic granules or powder

15 grams dried onion granules or powder

30 grams coarse unrefined sea salt

EQUIPMENT

Kitchen scale

Latex gloves

Spice grinder or mortar and pestle

Food processor or blender

1-quart or 1-liter wide-mouth glass jar

Canning funnel (optional)

Parchment paper or cheesecloth cut to the diameter of the jar

Fermentation lid

Fine-mesh sieve

Smaller bottles or jars with lids, for storage

Being third- and fourth-generation Californians, respectively, Mexican food is a mainstay in our diets, and no burrito or taco is complete without a stellar hot sauce to accompany it. The most iconic hot sauce of California has to be Pepper Plant, which holds a prominent place in our refrigerator and is an awesome addition to eggs, potato dishes, marinades, and of course any Mexican dish. Its mild spice and rich garlic flavor makes this pepper sauce ideal for those who don't want too much spice but still want to add flavor (and a hint of spice) to any dish. We thought it was only proper to include our version of this iconic California pepper sauce in our list of mashes and hot sauces. And since Pepper Plant is produced in the "garlic capital of the world," Gilroy, California (very near our production facility), garlic figures prominently in our version.

My longtime girlfriend, Amy, loves Pepper Plant above all other hot sauces. If we find ourselves having breakfast out and they don't have Pepper Plant for her eggs and potatoes, we aren't likely to be returning to that restaurant anytime soon. This one is for you, Amy! —Shane

1. Wash and sanitize all your fermentation equipment, including a knife and cutting board, and set aside to air-dry.

2. Toast the coriander and cumin in a dry skillet over medium heat until they turn golden. Transfer to a small plate and let cool, then grind in a spice grinder or using a mortar and pestle.

3. Put the peppers in your food processor or blender; add the ground coriander and cumin, the water, chipotle, fresh garlic and garlic granules, onion granules, and salt; and process for 2 to 3 minutes, until the mash is smooth. (The larger pepper pieces will often float to the top of the mash in the food processor, so alternate running the motor and pulsing to be sure they're incorporated.) Open the processor, being careful not to inhale the pepper fumes, and scrape down the sides of the processor bowl with a spatula. Process for 1 to 2 minutes more, until the mash is quite liquid.

4. Transfer the pepper mash to the jar along with any liquid (a canning funnel is useful here and helps to minimize spillage), pushing it down with a spatula or wooden spoon to remove any air pockets and leaving 1 inch of headspace. Place the parchment paper or cheesecloth in the jar over the mash (the mash should be completely covered).

CONTINUED >

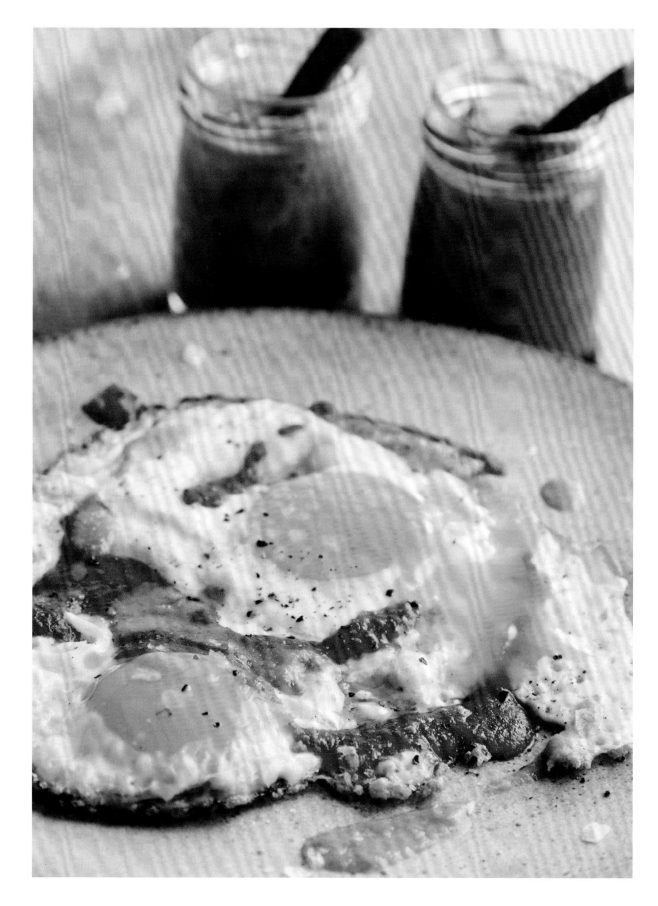

5. Seal the jar with the fermentation lid. Place the sealed jar on a plate or in a bowl to catch any liquid displaced through the airlock during fermentation.

6. Ferment the pepper mash in a cool place away from direct sunlight (2 months at 64°F is ideal—see the chart on page 185). Keep an eye on the mash through the first 2 weeks— if it loses enough liquid during the first phase of fermentation that the top layer is exposed, top it off with brine (see Fermenter's Notes, page 181). Also, keep an eye on the airlock to make sure it never runs dry, cleaning it and refilling with fresh water as needed. Taste the pepper mash after 1 month to determine if the flavor is to your liking. If it's not, reseal the jar and leave to ferment for another month, then taste again.

7. When the pepper mash is to your liking, strain it through a fine-mesh sieve into a bowl, the solids out using a fine sieve. Press pressing down on the mash solids with a wooden spoon to extract as much liquid as possible. (reserve the spent solids to make a pepper seasoning, if you like—see Note, page 185). Transfer the liquid hot sauce into smaller bottles or jars, seal, and move to refrigeration. It will last store in the refrigerator. It will keep for at least 10 months in refrigeration.

SRIRACHA

MAKES 1 QUART

900 grams coarsely chopped red jalapeños or serrano peppers, including seeds

50 grams garlic powder

30 grams coarse unrefined sea salt

20 grams agar-agar powder

EQUIPMENT

Kitchen scale

Latex gloves

Food processor or blender

1-quart or 1-liter wide-mouth glass jar

Canning funnel (optional)

Parchment paper or cheesecloth cut to the diameter of the jar

Fermentation lid

Smaller bottles or jars with lids, for storage

Originally from Thailand, sriracha is typically made with red jalapeño peppers, garlic powder, vinegar, sugar, salt, and—here's where things go wrong for us—preservatives and thickeners. Making your own allows you to choose the best-quality ingredients without sacrificing flavor, and homemade sriracha keeps for months in the fridge, so there's no need for preservatives.

1. Wash and sanitize all your fermentation equipment, including a knife and cutting board, and set aside to air-dry.

2. Put the peppers in the food processor or blender, add the garlic powder and salt, and process for 2 to 3 minutes, until the mash is smooth. (The larger pepper pieces will often float to the top of the mash in the food processor, so alternate running the motor and pulsing to be sure they're incorporated.) Open the processor, being careful not to inhale the pepper fumes, and scrape down the sides of the processor bowl with a spatula. Process for 1 to 2 minutes more, until the mash is quite liquid.

3. Transfer the pepper mash to the jar along with any liquid (a canning funnel is useful here and helps to minimize spillage), pushing it down with a spatula or wooden spoon to remove any air pockets and leaving 1 inch of headspace. Place the parchment paper or cheesecloth in the jar over the mash (the mash should be completely covered). Seal the jar with the fermentation lid. Place the sealed jar on a plate or in a bowl to catch any liquid displaced through the airlock during fermentation.

4. Ferment the pepper mash in a cool place away from direct sunlight (2 months at 64°F is ideal—see the chart on page 185). Keep an eye on the mash through the first 2 weeks— if it loses enough liquid during the first phase of fermentation that the top layer is exposed, top it off with brine (see Fermenter's Notes, page 181). Also, keep an eye on the airlock to make sure it never runs dry, cleaning it and refilling with fresh water as needed. Taste the pepper mash after 1 month to determine if the flavor is to your liking. If it's not, reseal the jar and leave to ferment for another month, then taste again. When the pepper mash is to your liking, transfer it to a blender, add the agar-agar, and blend into a thick sauce. Transfer the sauce into bottles or jars, seal, and store in the refrigerator for up to 1 year, though it will likely last much longer.

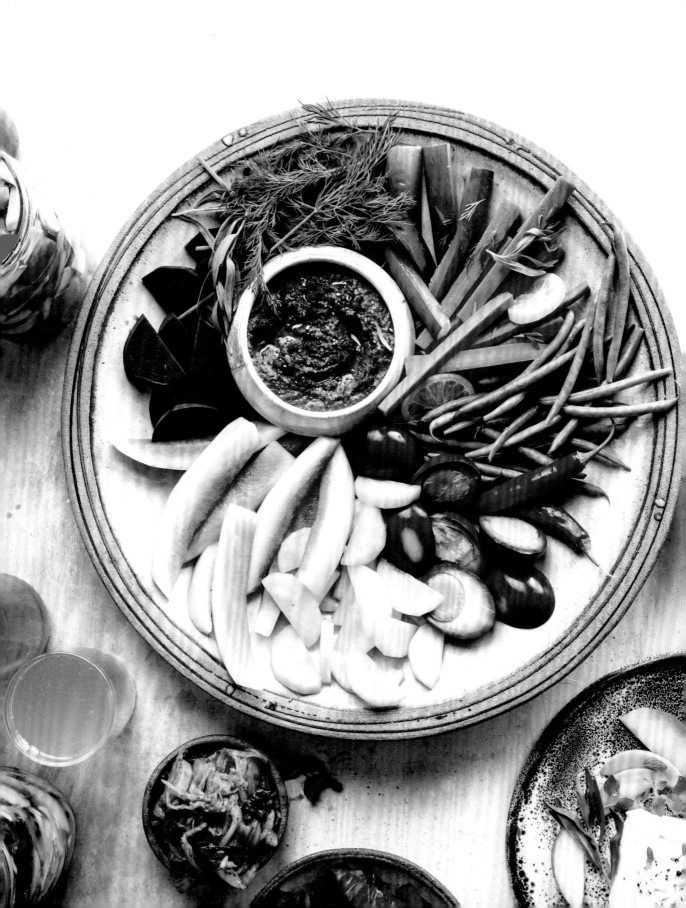

Brined Ferments

Brining is often confused with the term *pickling*, which actually comes from the Dutch word *pekel*, which means "brine." Most of us associate pickling with a vinegar, so for the sake of clarity, we're using the term "brined" to refer to fermentation in a water-and-salt solution. This method is recommended for low-moisture vegetables that may not produce enough liquid to make a natural brine when dry-salted, or when you want to ferment a whole vegetable. Brining can also be very effective for keeping yeasts and alcohol at bay when fermenting fruits. The strength of the brine can vary considerably depending on what you're fermenting. Cucumber pickles (see page 246), for instance, require a fairly salty brine to counteract the vegetable's natural softening enzymes. The ferments in this section generally utilize lower-salt solutions.

FERMENTER'S NOTES

Produce: Selecting the freshest vegetables and fruits possible means you'll start your ferment off on the right foot with a good dose of naturally occurring lactic acid bacteria (LAB), found on the skins. For this reason, we recommend lightly rinsing rather than peeling produce. Older produce not only has less lactic acid bacteria, but may also bring mold and yeast into play, which can potentially ruin your ferment. For mixed vegetable medleys, remember to choose produce with similar density and texture so they're ready at the same time. We've selected the Taco Bar Mix (page 210) as our master recipe because it showcases fairly ideal vegetables that ferment well together, including onions. Although they are softer than the other vegetables in the mix, their tight cellular structure means they hold up well.

Produce weight, density, and volume vary considerably. Cauliflower, for instance takes up a good deal more space in a crock or jar than, say, sliced radishes. We've taken this into account when designing these recipes so you don't have to worry about figuring out the ratio of solids to brine. When you're ready to create your own recipes, we've found that as a general rule, 45% solids to 55% brine works for most vegetables and fruits, though you may have to do a little experimenting to get the ratio just right.

Water: Good-quality spring or well water is ideal for brining because it's full of minerals that the bacteria like. The vegetables and fruit you'll be brining also contain plenty of these nutrients, though, so filtered or distilled water works just fine.

Salt: Generally speaking, the acceptable range for brine strength is between 3 and 5% salt by weight to water, though you will see some ferments that occasionally fall outside of this range. Most of our brined recipes are made using a brine strength of 3%. This is at the lower end of the accepted salt range, but we are able to get away with a lower salt percentage because we are using a starter culture (see page 208). We have opted for a 4% brine for some of our recipes that contain fruit or vegetables with higher sugar content, in order to avoid the formation of alcohol. In warmer temperatures, which favor the growth of yeast, the brine strength can be increased to as high as 5 or even 6% to slow down the fermentation process and favor LAB. Although it seems like these brines are fairly salty, think about it like this: if you're using 50% water and 50% solids, a 4% brine is roughly equivalent to the 2% salt in a dry-salted ferment, like kraut. We would not advise you to go any lower than 3% brine, even in colder climates.

Brine: These recipes are designed to make extra brine, which should be reserved and stored in the refrigerator, where it will keep for seven to ten days. This brine can be used if you lose some of the brine through the airlock or lid during the fermentation process. If this happens, open the jar, add the replacement brine, leaving 2 inches of headspace, and reseal (leave the jar open only as long as it takes to add the brine, to avoid introducing unwanted yeasts and molds). During the first five to seven days, gas (CO_2) is produced, which can cause the brine to be expelled through the airlock, potentially dropping the brine level below the vegetables. If you add replacement brine too soon, it will just be expelled by the gases, too, so wait until the end of this first phase before adding more brine. The exposed vegetables are protected by a layer of CO_2 during this phase and generally will not deteriorate. You'll know this phase is complete when the brine stops bubbling.

Keeping your vegetables and fruits submerged in brine during and after the fermentation process is key to avoiding the growth of yeasts and molds. In dry-salted ferments, you can just scrape them off, but with brined ferments, the yeasts and molds can penetrate the brine and affect the vegetables, ruining the ferment (see page 83 for more on this). We recommend a number of options for keeping foods submerged on pages 47 to 50.

Culture: All the brined ferments in this chapter use basic kraut brine as a starter culture, but you can use another starter if you prefer (see page 64 for other options). We do this to give the ferment a head start, and to keep yeast from outcompeting the LAB; yeast, if allowed to proliferate, can result in off flavors and the formation of alcohol. Culturing also means that you can use less salt, which we think makes for better-tasting ferments. And finally, by adding kraut brine, you're getting the added benefits of all the wild microflora it brings to the party. You can also very easily skip the starter and wild ferment your produce using their natural microflora instead (see page 64 for more on wild ferments). If you take this route, we advise that you increase the brine strength to 4 to 5% salt, bearing in mind that this will affect the flavor of the ferment.

Fermenting: Ferment in a cool place away from direct sunlight for the time prescribed in each recipe. It is sometimes acceptable to opt for a shorter fermentation time if you really like how the ferment tastes at the stage; however, it should be noted that if there are residual sugars in the vegetables, the ferment may become slightly effervescent in the refrigerator. In some recipes, this can be quite nice; in others, it's off-putting. Generally speaking, it's better to let the ferment go the full recommended time.

Tasting: When the time comes to taste your brined ferment, remove the lid and use a clean, nonreactive utensil to pull out a sample, then immediately replace the lid in order keep airborne microbes out. You'll know the ferment is ready when it tastes pleasingly tart, but not bracingly sour. The texture of the fermented vegetable or fruit should be softer than it was raw, but not mushy. The brine typically gets cloudy as the ferment progresses. This is perfectly normal and, along with taste, is a good way to tell that your ferment is nearly ready.

Storage: We recommend transferring all brined ferments to smaller jars (pints are perfect) for storage because they keep longer if left undisturbed until you're ready to eat them. Make sure to evenly divide the vegetables and brine among the jars, and to keep the vegetables submerged. If some of the vegetables still want to float, use the weight you used for fermentation to keep them submerged in the brine. If you end up short on brine you can use the reserved brine or make additional brine for packing.

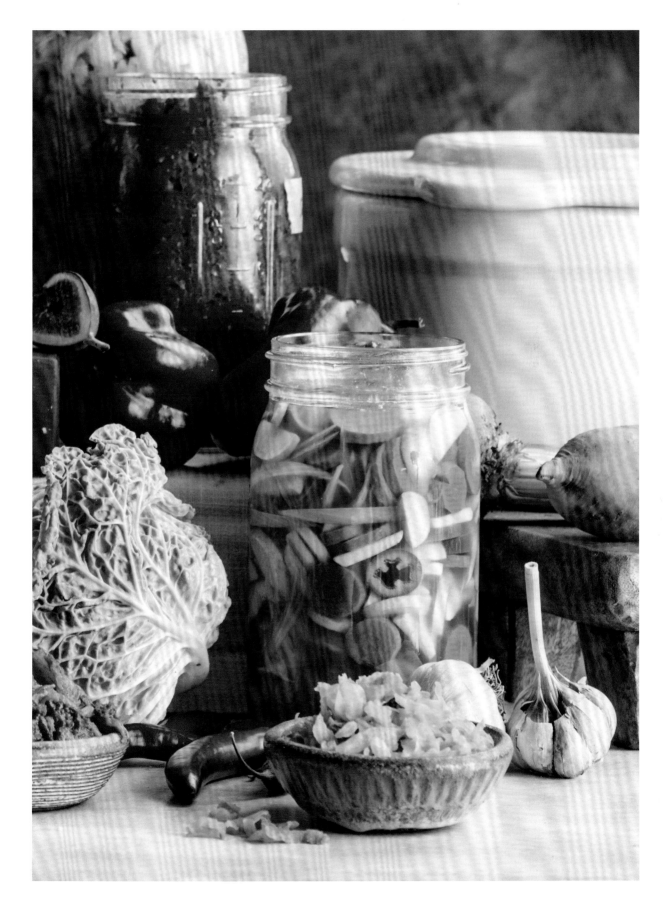

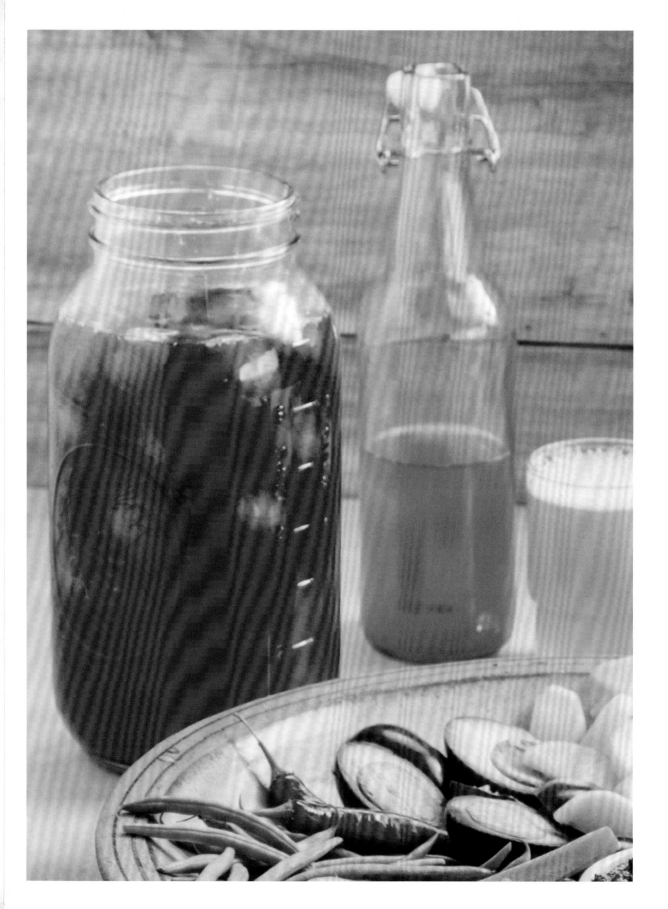

RUBY RADISHES

MAKES ½ GALLON

970 milliliters distilled or spring water

30 grams unrefined sea salt

900 grams whole red radishes, lightly rinsed

100 milliliters natural brine from Basic Kraut (page 92) or from store-bought plain kraut

EQUIPMENT

Kitchen scale

½-gallon or 2-liter wide-mouth glass jar

Weight

Fermentation lid

We think this is one of those simple ferments you should always have on hand in the refrigerator for a quick nosh or a crudité platter, or to slice and add to a salad. Fermenting mellows radishes, and their sturdy texture stands up nicely to the process. After a few days of soaking in brine, a magical transition takes place: the radishes' ruby red coats slip off and turn the brine a brilliant reddish pink, leaving behind little rose-colored orbs. The brine is simply divine and can be a playful, tinted addition to any number of dishes. Pink egg salad? Why not?

1. Wash and sanitize all your fermentation equipment, including a knife and cutting board, and set aside to air-dry.

2. Make a salt brine by bringing 300 milliliters of the water to just under a boil in a small saucepan. Remove from the heat, add the salt, and stir well until all the salt has dissolved. Add the remaining 670 milliliters room-temperature water to the hot brine to cool it down; set aside.

3. Put the radishes in the jar. Pour the kraut brine into the jar over the radishes. Pour the salt brine into the jar, leaving about 2 inches of headspace. Reserve the extra salt brine in a small jar in the refrigerator to use as needed.

4. Place the weight in the jar on top of the radishes and press down until the radishes are completely submerged in the brine. Seal the jar with the fermentation lid. Place the sealed jar on a plate or in a bowl to catch any liquid displaced through the airlock during fermentation.

5. Ferment the radishes in a cool place away from direct sunlight (3 weeks at 64°F is ideal—see the chart on page 211). If, after the first 5 to 7 days, the level of the brine drops below the radishes, add reserved brine as needed (see Fermenter's Notes, page 207). Taste the radishes after 2 weeks to determine if the flavor and sourness are to your liking. If they're not sour enough, reseal the jar and let them ferment for another week, then taste again. When the radishes are to your liking, replace the fermentation lid with a regular lid, seal, and store in the refrigerator for up to 6 months.

JACK'S PICKLED PEPPERS

970 milliliters distilled or
spring water

30 grams dried New Mexico
chiles

30 grams unrefined sea salt

1 teaspoon dried oregano

1 teaspoon dried thyme

450 grams whole fresh jalapeños

450 grams whole fresh serrano
peppers

100 milliliters natural brine from
Basic Kraut (page 92) or from
store-bought plain kraut

EQUIPMENT

Kitchen scale

½-gallon or 2-liter wide-mouth
glass jar

Weight

Fermentation lid

These pickled peppers are dedicated to my grandfather Jack Peterson, who had a huge influence on me becoming the man I am today. He taught me how to compost. With his prolific garden, he inspired me at an early age to get my hands in the soil. And most of all, he taught me to love nature. I'll never forget the moment when he plucked a turnip from the ground, pulled out his pocket knife, and carved it up. He handed me the white flesh, and with that bite, I was transformed forever. He was constantly cracking jokes and he regularly sported a mile-wide shit-eating grin. I only wish I had spent more time in his garden with him.

Grandpa Jack grew up on a 300-acre cotton ranch in Las Cruces, New Mexico. He was short in stature, but fast as the night is long, and dark in nature and complexion owing to his Chickasaw roots. As the story goes, Jack, being a transplant to California with his siblings and parents still tending the ranch, looked forward to his annual package from home, consisting of a case of his brother's spicy pickled peppers, more than anything in the world. "Now that's a Mexican pickle, boy," he used to say upon tasting and sharing his beloved pickled peppers (he called most everyone younger than himself "boy"). One year, when my father was very young, Jack thought it would be funny to give him one of those pickled peppers. The way my father tells it, Jack thought it was hilarious, and as my father suffered through the pain, Jack laughed and laughed and laughed. Jack just may have poisoned him for life with that capsaicin crudité, because my father, Steven, will literally begin perspiring at the thought of spicy foods. I inherited both Jack's love of spicy foods and his proclivity for mischievous practical jokes. This one is for you, Jack. —Shane

1. Wash and sanitize all your fermentation equipment, including a knife and cutting board, and set aside to air-dry.

2. Make a chile brine by bringing 300 milliliters of the water to a boil in a small saucepan. Remove from the heat and add the dried New Mexico chiles. Cover and let soak for 20 minutes. Strain the soaking liquid through a fine-mesh sieve set over a medium bowl, pressing down on the chiles with a wooden spoon to extract as much liquid as possible; discard the chiles. Add the salt to the chile soaking liquid and stir until it has dissolved. Add the remaining 670 milliliters room-temperature water to the hot brine to cool it down; set aside.

3. Put the oregano and thyme in the jar. Pack the jalapeños and serranos into the jar (no need to stem them). Pour the kraut brine into the jar over the peppers. Pour the chile brine into the jar, leaving about 2 inches of headspace. Reserve the extra chile brine in a small jar in the refrigerator to use as needed.

4. Place the weight in the jar on top of the peppers and press down until the peppers are completely submerged in the brine. Seal the jar with the fermentation lid. Place the sealed jar on a plate or in a bowl to catch any liquid displaced through the airlock during fermentation.

5. Ferment the peppers in a cool place away from direct sunlight (3 weeks at 64°F is ideal—see the chart on page 211). If, after the first 5 to 7 days, the level of the brine drops below the peppers, add reserved brine as needed (see Fermenter's Notes, page 207). Taste the peppers after 2 weeks to determine if the flavor and sourness are to your liking. If they're not sour enough, reseal the jar and let them ferment for another week, then taste again. When the peppers are to your liking, replace the fermentation lid with a regular lid, seal, and store in the refrigerator for up to 6 months.

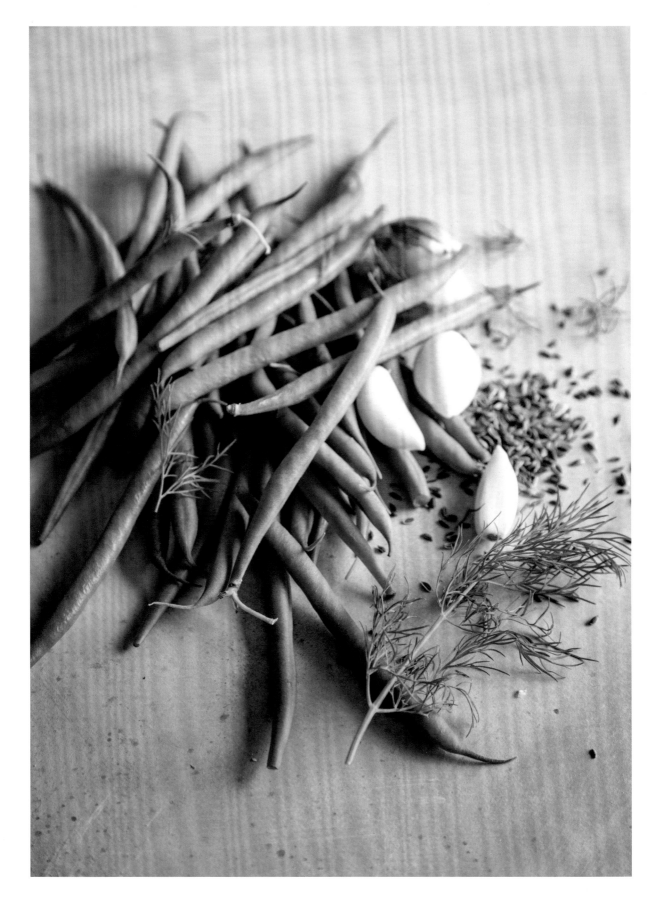

DILLY BEANS

MAKES ½ GALLON

970 milliliters distilled or spring water

30 grams unrefined sea salt

40 grams whole peeled garlic cloves

10 grams dried dill seed

840 grams trimmed fresh green beans, lightly rinsed

10 grams fresh dill sprigs

100 milliliters natural brine from Basic Kraut (page 92) or from store-bought plain kraut

EQUIPMENT

Kitchen scale

½-gallon or 2-liter wide-mouth glass jar

Weight

Fermentation lid

No other traditional vinegar pickle translates as well to a fermented version as dilly beans do. We wanted to create a simple and very dill-forward recipe, so we doubled down and used both fresh and dried dill. Fresh dill brings lemony, anise notes to the party and is complemented by the dill seeds, which are reminiscent of caraway (which can be substituted for the dill seed).

Kids tend to love these beans straight out of the jar or with something alongside for dipping. The brine is a stunning addition to potato and egg salads, and a tablespoon will elevate your dill dip to the next level. Salad dressing will also benefit from a tablespoon or two of the dilly brine.

1. Wash and sanitize all your fermentation equipment, including a knife and cutting board, and set aside to air-dry.

2. Make a salt brine by bringing 300 milliliters of the water to just under a boil in a small saucepan. Remove from the heat, add the salt, and stir well until all the salt has dissolved. Add the remaining 670 milliliters room-temperature water to the hot brine to cool it down; set aside.

3. Put the garlic and dill seed in the jar. Pack the green beans upright in the jar, along with the fresh dill sprigs, fitting them among the green beans as you go. Pour the kraut brine into the jar over the green beans. Pour the salt brine into the jar, leaving about 2 inches of headspace. Reserve the extra salt brine in a small jar in the refrigerator to use as needed.

4. Place the weight in the jar on top of the green beans and press down until the green beans are completely submerged in the brine. Seal the jar with the fermentation lid. Place the sealed jar on a plate or in a bowl to catch any liquid displaced through the airlock during fermentation.

5. Ferment the green beans in a cool place away from direct sunlight (3 weeks at 64°F is ideal—see the chart on page 211). If, after the first 5 to 7 days, the level of the brine drops below the green beans, add reserved brine as needed (see Fermenter's Notes, page 207). Taste the green beans after 2 weeks to determine if the flavor and sourness are to your liking. If they're not sour enough, reseal the jar and let them ferment for another week, then taste again. When the dilly beans are to your liking, replace the fermentation lid with a regular lid, seal, and store in the refrigerator for up to 6 months.

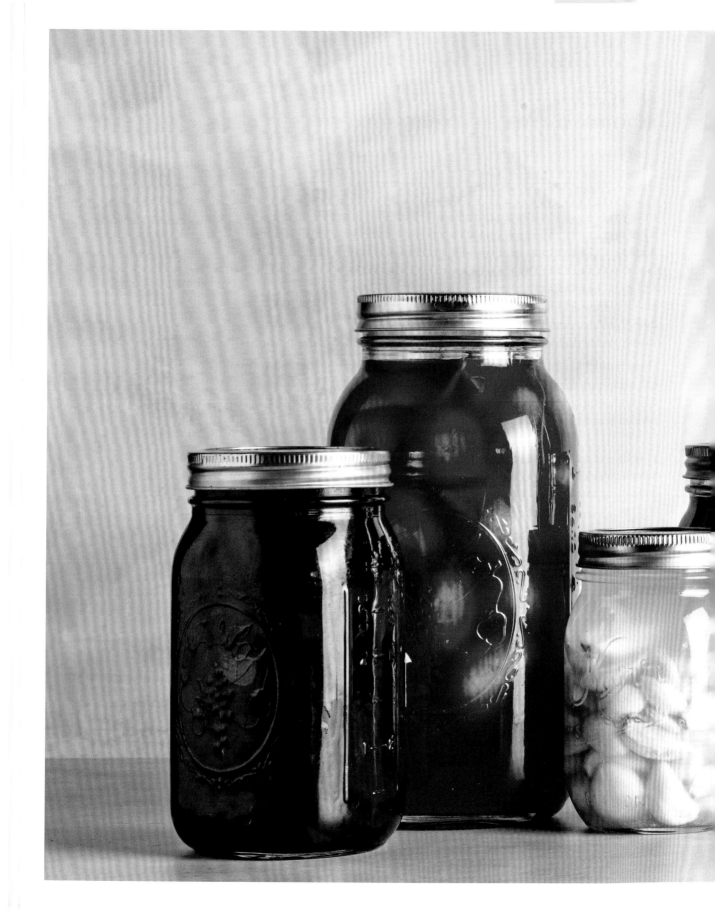

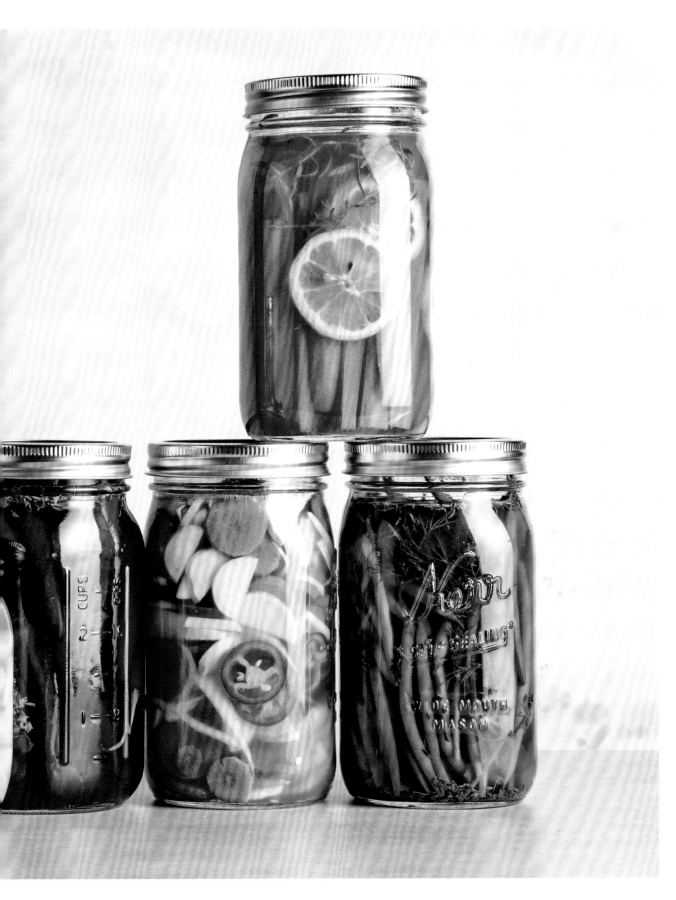

970 milliliters distilled or
spring water

30 grams unrefined sea salt

50 grams thinly sliced
green garlic or whole
peeled garlic cloves

800 grams trimmed asparagus,
lightly rinsed

2 lemons (about 50 grams total),
well rinsed: 1 halved, 1 sliced
into rounds

100 milliliters natural brine from
Basic Kraut (page 92) or from
store-bought plain kraut

EQUIPMENT

Kitchen scale

½-gallon or 2-liter wide-mouth
glass jar

Weight

Fermentation lid

ASPARAGUS
with Green Garlic and Lemon

Every spring, we are inspired to ferment those gangly stalks of asparagus as they start to pop up at farmers' markets. We've noticed that once fermented, the thinner asparagus spears can be delicate, so use slightly thicker spears if they're available.

Fermented asparagus stalks make an enticing addition to a crudité platter, or try chopping it up and adding it to egg salad for a delightful spring sandwich or salad topping. For a playful and probiotic Bloody Mary, add a jigger of the brine, and use a fermented asparagus stalk as a stir stick. We can't think of a better way to celebrate spring!

1. Wash and sanitize all your fermentation equipment, including a knife and cutting board, and set aside to air-dry.

2. Make a salt brine by bringing 300 milliliters of the water to just under a boil in a small saucepan. Remove from the heat, add the salt, and stir well until all the salt has dissolved. Add the remaining 670 milliliters room-temperature water to the hot brine to cool it down; set aside.

3. Put the garlic in the jar. Pack the asparagus spears upright into the jar. Juice the halved lemon directly into the jar and pack the lemon slices between the side of the jar and the asparagus. Pour the kraut brine into the jar over the asparagus. Pour the salt brine into the jar, leaving about 2 inches of headspace. Reserve the extra salt brine in a small jar in the refrigerator to use as needed.

4. Place the weight in the jar on top of the asparagus and press down until the asparagus is completely submerged in the brine. Seal the jar with the fermentation lid. Place the sealed jar on a plate or in a bowl to catch any liquid displaced through the airlock during fermentation.

5. Ferment the brined asparagus in a cool place away from direct sunlight (3 weeks at 64°F is ideal—see the chart on page 211). If, after the first 5 to 7 days, the level of the brine drops below the asparagus, add reserved brine as needed (see Fermenter's Notes, page 207). Taste the asparagus after 2 weeks to determine if the flavor and sourness are to your liking. If it's not sour enough, reseal the jar and let it ferment for another week, then taste again. When the asparagus is to your liking, replace the fermentation lid with a regular lid, seal, and store in the refrigerator for up to 6 months.

LEMON-TARRAGON CARROT STICKS

MAKES ½ GALLON

970 milliliters distilled or spring water

30 grams unrefined sea salt

820 grams sliced carrots (½-inch-thick spears), lightly rinsed

2 lemons, preferably Meyer (about 60 grams total), well rinsed: 1 halved, 1 sliced into rounds

20 grams fresh tarragon leaves

100 milliliters natural brine from Basic Kraut (page 92) or from store-bought plain kraut

EQUIPMENT

Kitchen scale

½-gallon or 2-liter wide-mouth glass jar

Weight

Fermentation lid

One might think that any ol' carrot would do for a fermentation crock, but there is a world of difference in flavor and nutrition between organic farmers' market carrots and that five-pound bag from the produce aisle. Several studies, cited in respected journals, found that organically grown carrots contain significantly more vitamins, minerals, and antioxidants such as polyphenols.[1] Like, a lot more. Maybe this is why carrots don't really taste like, well, carrots anymore, and why they don't behave as well in the crock. Fermented carrots are susceptible to yeast, which is not harmful, but can produce off flavors in the finished ferment. We've found that those gorgeous, gem-colored, skinny carrots from the farmers' market produce consistently good-tasting fermented carrots with no funky finish. Making sure the carrots remain submerged in their brine is also important.

We add tarragon at the beginning of the ferment, but it is a delicate herb that can lose some of its flavor during fermentation, so we sometimes chop up a bit more and add it to the finished brine. To avoid the bitterness that can sometimes occur when fermenting lemons, we recommend using Meyer lemons or a lemon with less pith (the bitter culprit), if possible.

These carrot sticks are wonderful on a crudité platter or simply as a grab-and-go snack. And don't waste the carrot tops. Use them as you would an herb, such as finely chopped in tabouli or other salads. They are also quite good in hummus, which you could then drag your fermented carrot sticks through.

CONTINUED >

1 Roddy Scheer and Doug Moss, "Dirt Poor: Have Fruits and Vegetables Become Less Nutritious?" Earthtalk, *Scientific American*, www.scientificamerican.com/article/soil-depletion-and-nutrition-loss; M. Barański, D. Srednicka-Tober, N. Volakakis, et al., "Higher Anitoxidant and Lower Cadmium Concentrations and Lower incidence of Pesticide Residues in Organically Grown Crops: A Systematic Literature Review and Meta-Analyses," *British Journal of Nutrition* 112, no. 5 (Sept. 14, 2014): 794–811, www.ncbi.nlm.nih.gov/pubmed/24968103; "Carrots," What's on My Food?, www.whatsonmyfood.org/food.jsp?food=CR.

1. Wash and sanitize all your fermentation equipment and set aside to air-dry.

2. Make a salt brine by bringing 150 milliliters of the water to just under a boil in a small saucepan. Remove from the heat, add the salt, and stir well until all the salt has dissolved. Add the remaining 335 milliliters room-temperature water to the hot brine to cool it down; set aside.

3. Put the garlic in the jar. Pour the kraut brine into the jar over the garlic. Pour the salt brine into the jar, leaving about 2 inches of headspace. Reserve the extra salt brine in a small jar in the refrigerator to use as needed.

4. Place the weight in the jar on top of the garlic and press down until the garlic is completely submerged in the brine. Seal the jar with the fermentation lid. Place the sealed jar on a plate or in a bowl to catch any liquid displaced through the airlock during fermentation.

5. Ferment the garlic in a cool place away from direct sunlight (3 weeks at 64°F is ideal—see the chart on page 211). If, after the first 5 to 7 days, the level of the brine drops below the garlic, add reserved brine as needed (see Fermenter's Notes, page 207). Taste the garlic after 2 weeks to determine if the flavor and sourness are to your liking. If it's not sour enough, reseal the jar and let it ferment for another week, then taste again. When the garlic is to your liking, replace the fermentation lid with a regular lid, seal, and store in the refrigerator for up to 6 months.

Note: Have you ever seen blue garlic? The acidity in pickling and fermenting can cause garlic to release a compound called isoallin, which can give it a blue-green tint. This is not a frequent occurrence, but if it does happen, worry not—your garlic is perfectly safe to eat and its flavor won't be affected.

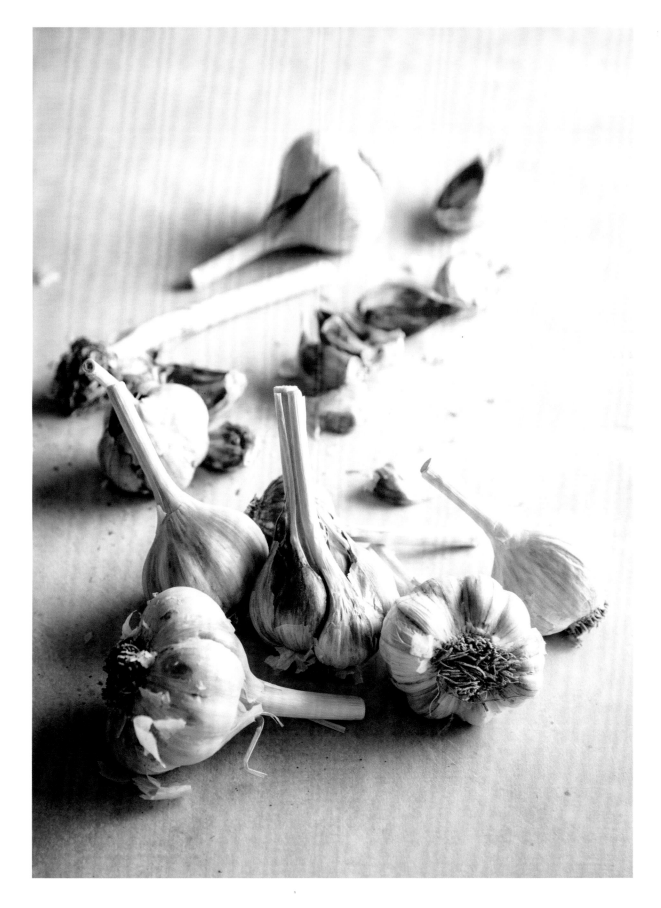

960 milliliters distilled or
spring water

40 grams unrefined sea salt

300 grams sliced red bell
peppers (1-inch-wide strips)

300 grams sliced yellow bell
peppers (1-inch-wide strips)

300 grams sliced orange bell
peppers (1-inch-wide strips)

1 teaspoon dried oregano

1 teaspoon dried thyme

100 milliliters natural brine from
Basic Kraut (page 92) or from
store-bought plain kraut

EQUIPMENT

Kitchen scale

½-gallon or 2-liter wide-mouth
glass jar

Weight

Fermentation lid

SWEET ITALIAN MIXED PEPPERS

We wanted to create a fermented version of the marinated roasted peppers found on Italian antipasto platters, and after several iterations, landed on this recipe, which we think is every bit as good as the original. In addition to their great flavor, the prep time is faster, too—no need to peel the peppers as you typically would before marinating, because the skins become silky soft in the crock. We make big batches when red, orange, and yellow bells peppers are in season (they can be expensive out of season), and have found that they keep for months in the refrigerator.

Peppers are part of the nightshade family, and as much I love them, I have to eat nightshades sparingly because I find they make me achy. However, I've noticed that I can eat relatively large amounts of fermented nightshades without any problem. I have no scientific evidence to back this up, but I think something is definitely happening in the crock that neutralizes the alkaloids.

My favorite movie of all time is *Moonstruck*. In the last scene, Olympia Dukakis makes what we in our family call "*Moonstruck* eggs": I carve a hole in the middle of a piece of bread, put it in a pan, crack an egg into it, cook the egg over-easy, and serve the eggy toast with marinated sweet red bell peppers. Aside from serving these peppers with *Moonstruck* eggs, one of our favorite ways to eat them is with buffalo mozzarella, smothered in good-quality olive oil. They're also delicious on sandwiches and in pasta dishes. —Kathryn

1. Wash and sanitize all your fermentation equipment, including a large bowl, knife, and cutting board, and set aside to air-dry.

2. Make a salt brine by bringing 300 milliliters of the water to just under a boil in a small saucepan. Remove from the heat, add the salt, and stir well until all the salt has dissolved. Add the remaining 670 milliliters room-temperature water to the hot brine to cool it down; set aside.

3. In the large bowl, combine the peppers, oregano, and thyme. Using clean hands, toss to combine. Transfer the peppers to the jar. (Alternatively, simply layer the peppers in the jar distributing the herbs as you go, one color after the next, which produces a beautiful effect.) Pour the kraut brine into the jar over the peppers. Pour the salt brine into the jar, leaving about 2 inches of headspace. Reserve the extra salt brine in a small jar in the refrigerator to use as needed.

4. Place the weight in the jar on top of the peppers and press down until the peppers are completely submerged in the brine. Seal the jar with the fermentation lid. Place the sealed jar on a plate or in a bowl to catch any liquid displaced through the airlock during fermentation.

5. Ferment the peppers in a cool place away from direct sunlight (10 days at 64°F is ideal—see the chart at right). If, after the first 5 to 7 days, the level of the brine drops below the peppers, add reserved brine as needed (see Fermenter's Notes, page 207). Taste the peppers after 1 week to determine if the flavor and sourness are to your liking. If they're not sour enough, reseal the jar and let them ferment for another week, then taste again. When the peppers are to your liking, replace the fermentation lid with a regular lid, seal, and store in the refrigerator for up to 6 months.

Fermentation Temperature & Time

Above 68°F
Ferment 7 days or less

65° to 68°F
Ferment 7 to 10 days

Ideal: 64°F
Ferment 10 days

60° to 63°F
Ferment 10 to 14 days

Below 60°F
Ferment 14 days or more

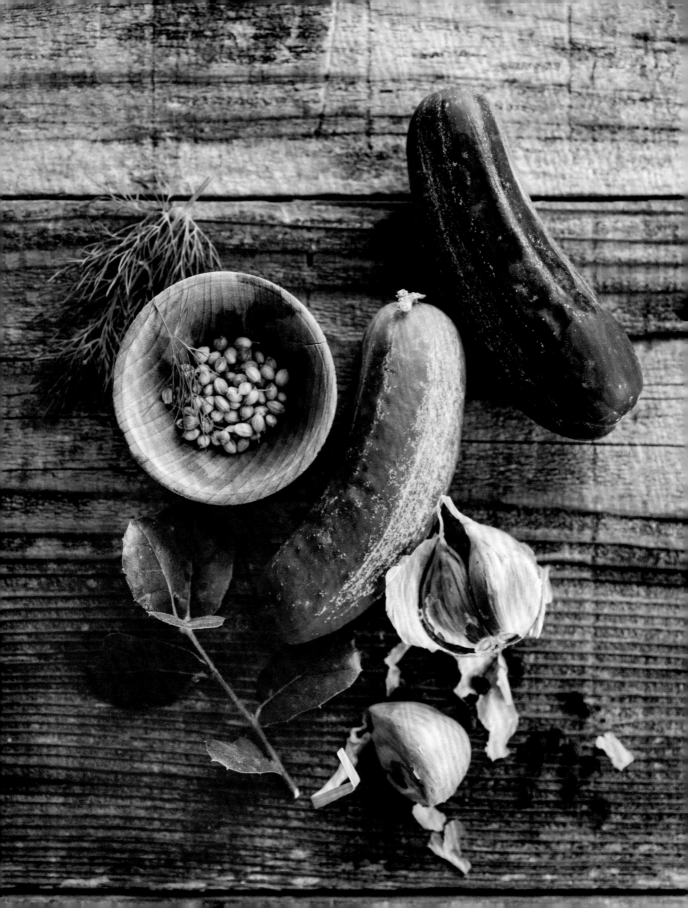

Cucumber Pickles

If I (Shane) had to choose one ferment that altered my perception and led me on the path to fermentation, it would have to be the cucumber pickle. When I began homesteading in earnest in 2012, some of the first crops I planted, besides cover crops and pollinator plants, were serrano peppers for making hot sauce and cucumbers for making pickles. I devoted an entire bed to each, in hopes of harvesting a bumper crop to fill my crocks. I'll never forget the pure joy I experienced throughout the process. I would wake early each day before work and head to the garden to tend it and check on the progress of my cucumbers and peppers. Throughout the summer, as the cucumbers grew steadfast on their trellis, creating a wall of leaves, flowers, and little green cucumbers, I would harvest them at just the right size and they would soon be in crocks, soaking in a salty brine. There is truly nothing more rewarding than growing produce and transforming it through the art of fermentation. For those of you who don't have the space or time to grow your own cucumbers, not to worry—you can still make incredibly tasty and satisfying homemade pickles.

There is quite a lot of confusion when it comes to the term *pickle*, which is broadly used to describe the process of vinegar pickling as well as fermenting in a brine. As famed food scientist Harold McGee states in *On Food and Cooking*, "The pickle, a food preserved by the immersion in brine or a strong acid such as vinegar. Brines often encourage fermentation, and fermentation generates preservative acids, so the term 'pickle' is applied to both fermented and unfermented preparations of cucumbers and other foods." Industrial vinegar pickles are typically fermented in massive vats in a salt brine (called *brine stock* in the industry); that brine is then strained and the pickles heated to kill all microrganisms, and a flavored vinegar brine is added at time of bottling. One of the main advantages of this process is that the cucumbers retain their crunchy texture far longer than their fermented counterparts. Fermented cucumbers are still alive, so the deterioration of their cell wall pectins continues even in the refrigerator, whereas the pasteurization and acidification of the industrial version means they will keep for literally years at room temperature and still maintain the delicious crunch that is vital to a good pickle. As such, the pickle industry is alive and thriving—even though the microbes in those glass jars, neatly stacked in the grocery store aisles, are neither.

FERMENTER'S NOTES

Produce: Pickling cucumbers come in many different varieties and are mostly picked early, when they are still small and their seeds have yet to fully develop. Cucumbers are a summer crop, but the exact time of harvest will vary from year to year. Fresh pickling cucumbers can be hard to come by in grocery stores. If you can't grow them yourself and can't find them at the grocery store, your best bet is seeking out your local farmers' markets and asking the producers which variety of cucumbers they're growing, at what stage the cucumbers are picked, and of course when they will be in season. If, after trying these avenues, you simply can't find pickling cucumbers but still really want to try your hand at making pickles, you can substitute thin-skinned slicing cucumbers such as Persians. Also, try using Persian cucumbers or other slicing varieties for the recipes in this chapter that don't require you to leave the cucumber whole, such as our pickle chip recipes (see pages 253 and 254). Small pickling cucumbers really do produce the best pickles if you are fermenting them whole.

Cucumber flowers, which are sometimes still present on cucumbers when you buy them, contain a softening enzyme. Prior to making pickles, remove these flowers and scrub the flowering end of the cucumber with care, or you'll likely be eating (or rather, not eating) soft pickles. No one likes a soft pickle. (For more on this, see "Maintaining texture," page 244.)

Water: Good-quality spring or well water is ideal for brining because it's full of minerals that the bacteria like. The cucumbers you'll be pickling also contain plenty of these nutrients, though, so filtered or distilled water works just fine.

Salt: When discussing cucumber pickles, the terms *full sour* and *half sour* are commonly used to describe both salt content and fermentation time. Full-sour pickles are fermented in a brine with 5% to 8% salt by weight, and are left to ferment until fully sour. Half-sour pickles are typically fermented in a brine with 3.5% salt by weight, and are moved to the refrigerator before they get fully sour. (We've also heard of a "three-quarters sour," which would obviously lie somewhere in the middle, but

"Good ideas, like good pickles, are crisp, enduring, and devilishly hard to make."

—RUSHWORTH KIDDER

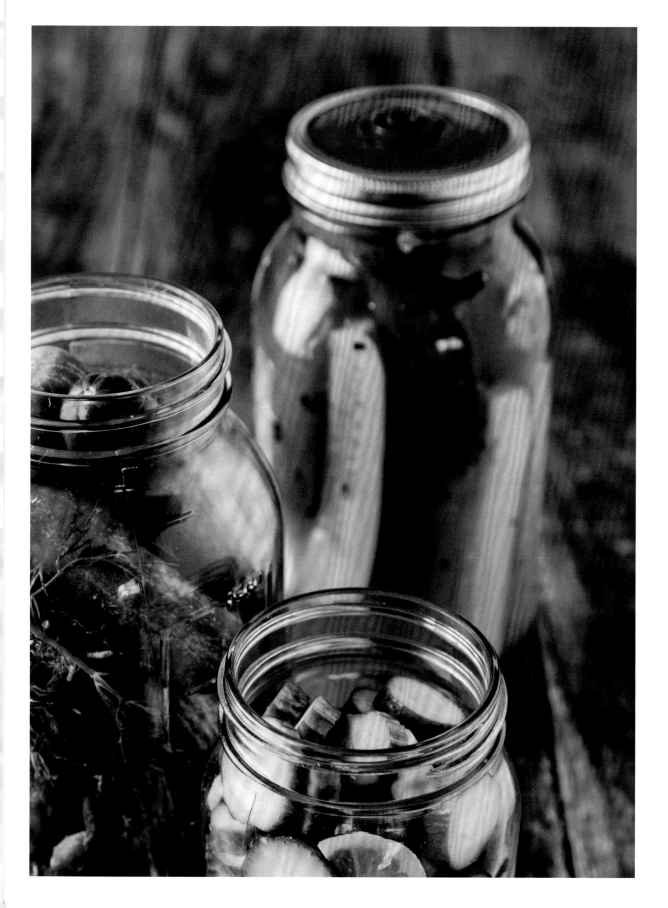

SMOKY TEA PICKLES

MAKES ½ GALLON

800 grams pickling cucumbers, ideally 3 to 5 inches long

965 milliliters distilled or spring water

35 grams unrefined sea salt

30 grams whole peeled garlic cloves (3 or 4 cloves)

2 teaspoons loose lapsang souchong tea

1 teaspoon whole black peppercorns

½ teaspoon ground chipotle chile

100 milliliters natural brine from Basic Kraut (page 92) or 100 grams Basic Kraut

EQUIPMENT

Kitchen scale

½-gallon or 2-liter wide-mouth glass jar

Weight

Fermentation lid

Robert's Tea Pickles from Linda Ziedrich's *Joy of Pickling* were so amazing that I started using the recipe regularly. The smokiness of the tea leaves takes the pickles to a new level of deliciousness and the tannins in tea help keep them crunchy. We've made a few changes to the original recipe and amplified the smoke with a little spicy heat from chipotle chiles. Most natural foods stores carry lapsang souchong, but it is also available online. —Kathryn

1. Wash and sanitize all your fermentation equipment, including a large bowl, knife, and cutting board, and set aside to air-dry. Fill the large bowl with ice and water.

2. Remove any flowers and scrape away any flower blossom residue from the ends of the cucumbers. As you work, put the cucumbers in the ice water to soak. Set aside to soak for 15 to 20 minutes.

3. Make a salt brine by bringing 300 milliliters of the water to just under a boil in a small saucepan. Remove from the heat, add the salt, and stir well until all the salt has dissolved. Add the remaining 665 milliliters room-temperature water to the hot brine to cool it down; set aside.

4. Add the garlic, tea leaves, peppercorns, and chile to the jar. Drain the cucumbers and tightly pack them upright in the jar. Pour the kraut brine and salt brine into the jar, leaving about 2 inches of headspace. Reserve the extra salt brine in a small jar in the refrigerator to use as needed.

5. Place the weight in the jar on top of the cucumbers and press down until the cucumbers are completely submerged in the brine. Seal the jar with the fermentation lid. Place the sealed jar on a plate or in a bowl to catch any liquid displaced through the airlock during fermentation.

6. Ferment the cucumbers in a cool, dark place away from direct sunlight (2 weeks at 64°F is ideal—see the chart on page 247). Taste the pickles after 1 week. If they aren't sour enough, reseal the jar and let them ferment for another week, then taste again. Fermented cucumbers should be tasted often, especially if they're being fermented in warmer temperatures. When the pickles are to your liking, replace the fermentation lid with a regular lid, seal, and store in the refrigerator for up to 6 months.

GINGER-TURMERIC PICKLE CHIPS

700 grams sliced Persian or
other slicing cucumbers

100 grams thinly sliced lemon
(from about 1 small lemon;
sliced into half-moons)

965 milliliters distilled or
spring water

35 grams unrefined sea salt

4 or 5 grape, oak, cherry,
or horseradish leaves, or
a combination (optional)

60 grams sliced peeled
fresh ginger

30 grams shredded peeled
fresh turmeric

1 teaspoon whole black
peppercorns, crushed

100 milliliters natural brine
from Basic Kraut (page 92)
or 100 grams Basic Kraut

EQUIPMENT

Kitchen scale

½-gallon or 2-liter wide-mouth
glass jars

Weight

Fermentation lid

All the goodness of ginger and the beauty of turmeric are found in this
scrumptious and nourishing pickle chip. To accentuate all the flavors, we've
included slices of lemon, which are nearly as good as the pickles—eat them
as is or use them whole on fish, chop them and add to salads, or blend them
into salad dressing. The fresh turmeric may tint your hands, so wear gloves
when handling it. Black pepper is also added to the mix to increase the
bioavailability of the turmeric and provide a nice little zing on the finish.

1. Wash and sanitize all your fermentation equipment, including a large
bowl, knife, and cutting board, and set
aside to air-dry. Fill the large bowl with
ice and water.

2. Trim the ends off the cucumbers,
adding them to the ice water as you go.
Set aside to soak for 15 to 20 minutes.

3. Make a salt brine by bringing
300 milliliters of the water to just under
a boil in a small saucepan. Remove
from the heat, add the salt, and stir
well until all the salt has dissolved.
Add the remaining 665 milliliters
room-temperature water to the hot
brine to cool it down; set aside.

4. If using the grape, oak, cherry, or
horseradish leaves, give them a quick
rinse and place them at the bottom
of the jar. Add the ginger, turmeric,
and peppercorns. Drain the cucumbers and slice them into ½-inch-thick
rounds. Pack them tightly into the jar.
Pour the kraut brine into the jar over
the cucumbers. Pour the salt brine
into the jar, leaving about 2 inches

of headspace. Reserve the extra salt
brine in a small jar in the refrigerator
to use as needed.

5. Place the weight in the jar on top
of the cucumbers and press down until
the cucumbers are completely submerged in the brine. Seal the jar with
the fermentation lid. Place the sealed
jar on a plate or in a bowl to catch any
liquid displaced through the airlock
during fermentation.

6. Ferment the cucumbers in a cool,
dark place away from direct sunlight
(2 weeks at 64°F is ideal—see the
chart on page 247). Taste the pickles after 1 week. If they aren't sour
enough, reseal the jar and let them
ferment for another week, then taste
again. Fermented cucumbers should
be tasted often, especially if they're
being fermented in warmer temperatures. When the pickles are to your
liking, replace the fermentation lid
with a regular lid, seal, and store in
the refrigerator for up to 6 months.

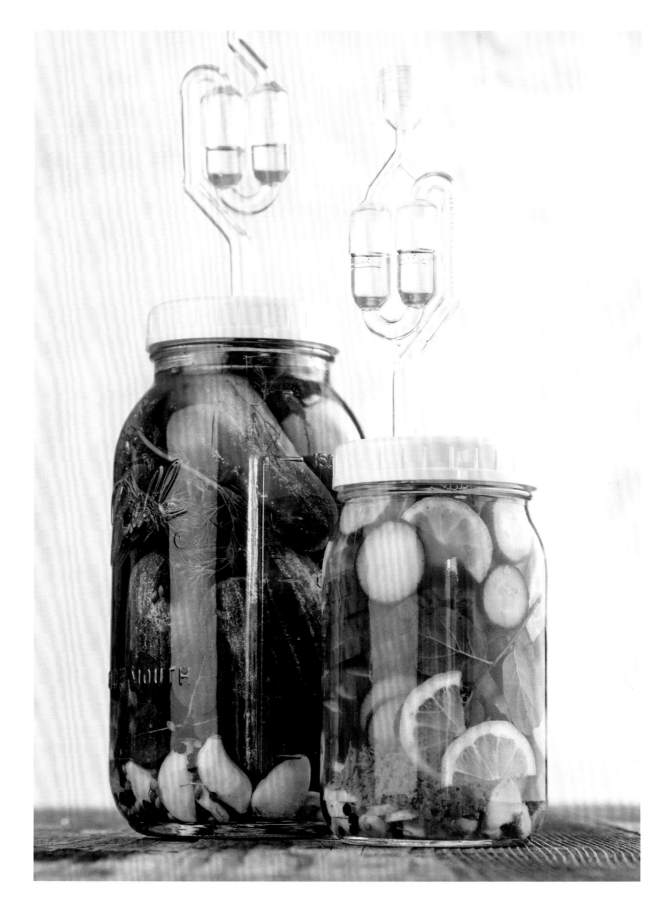

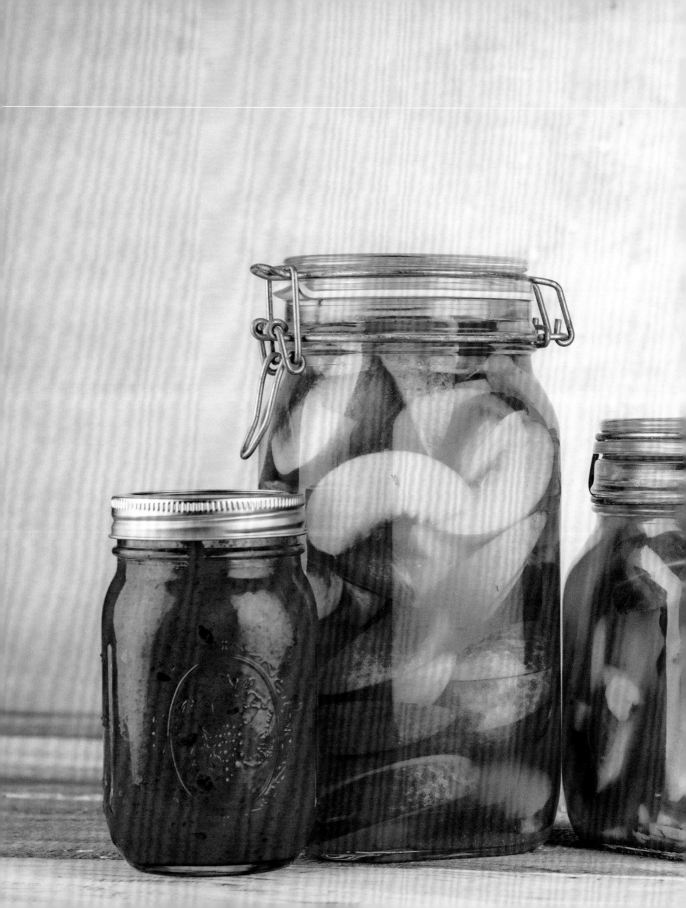

Fermented Fruit

960 milliliters distilled or spring water

40 grams unrefined sea salt

860 grams sliced peeled watermelon rinds (1-inch-wide by 4- to 6-inch-long strips; see Notes)

30 grams thinly sliced peeled fresh ginger (from one roughly 4-inch piece)

30 grams coarsely chopped candied ginger

10 grams fresh Makrut lime leaves (about 10)

¼ teaspoon red pepper flakes

100 milliliters natural brine from Basic Kraut (page 92) or from store-bought plain kraut

EQUIPMENT

Kitchen scale

½-gallon or 2-liter glass jar

Weight (optional)

Fermentation lid

SPICY GINGER–MAKRUT LIME WATERMELON RINDS

About 40 percent of the weight of a watermelon is in the rind, so rather than tossing it, why not make a scrumptious pickle? Most of the work is in the peeling, but that goes quickly once you find your rhythm. We prefer slicing the rinds into spears so they're easy to grab from the jar, but you can cut them any way you like. The rinds have a tendency to float, so make sure to weight them down so they stay submerged in the brine. Fresh Makrut lime leaves are so much better than dried; they're typically available at natural foods stores and gourmet grocers, but if you can't find them, substitute sliced lime in the same quantity.

The fermented rinds are fabulous chopped and added to a salad, or you can do as we do in our house and eat them straight out of the jar like a dill pickle.

1. Wash and sanitize all your fermentation equipment, including a knife and cutting board, and set aside to air-dry.

2. Make a salt brine by bringing 300 milliliters of the water to just under a boil in a small saucepan. Remove from the heat, add the salt, and stir well until all the salt has dissolved. Add the remaining 660 milliliters room-temperature water to the hot brine to cool it down; set aside.

3. Put the watermelon rinds in the jar, packing them in upright, adding both types of ginger, the lime leaves, and the red pepper flakes as you go. Pour the kraut brine into the jar over the rinds. Pour the salt brine into the jar, leaving about 2 inches of headspace. Reserve the extra salt brine in a small jar in the refrigerator to use as needed.

4. Place the weight in the jar on top of the rinds and press down until the rinds are completely submerged in the brine (see Notes). Seal the jar with the fermentation lid. Place the sealed jar on a plate or in a bowl to catch any liquid displaced through the airlock during fermentation.

5. Ferment the rinds in a cool place away from direct sunlight (7 days at 64°F is ideal—see the chart on page 260). Taste the rinds after 5 days to determine if the flavor and sourness are to your liking (remember to use a clean utensil and never double dip). If they're not sour enough, reseal the jar and let them ferment for another day or two, then taste again. When the rinds are to your liking, replace the fermentation lid with a regular lid, seal, and store in the refrigerator for up to 3 months.

Fermented Fruit

The first time we encountered fermented fruit was many years ago in Pasadena at Culture Club 101. The owner, Elaina Luther, although busy with many customers, took the time to let us sample all her goodies. Her whey-fermented jams were some of the best we'd ever tasted, but we still weren't clear why one would bother to ferment jam—and then it dawned on us: *It's the sugar, stupid!* Fermenting fruit of any kind converts some of the sugars into gut-loving microbes—or into alcohol. Let's back up a minute.

If you ferment fruit with either whey or kraut brine and you limit its time in the crock, you can successfully make mostly alcohol-free ferments. We say "mostly" because there may be a minuscule amount of alcohol in the finished ferment, but you'd be hard pressed to find it. In fact, barely detectable, tiny amounts of alcohol are found in many fermented foods and beverages, including kraut, kimchi, and kombucha, unless they've been pasteurized. That fresh-squeezed orange juice that's been in your refrigerator for a couple of days? Yep, tiny amounts of alcohol. For this reason we use kraut brine as a starter. It tends to produce a slightly tangier ferment, but is equally delicious and, generally speaking, produces less alcohol. An additional strategy is to remove as much yeast as possible from the skins of the fruit before fermenting. A good soak in distilled white vinegar or salted water kills most of the yeast responsible for forming alcohol.

So now that we have that out of the way, let's get back to the main reason to ferment fruit: the reduction of sugar and the addition of beneficial microbes. For some people, the high concentrations of sugars in fruit pump you up and then, a few hours later, throw you to the floor. Fermented fruit takes that experience down several notches by significantly reducing the sugar while leaving behind all the amazing health benefits. And who doesn't want less sugar in their diet?

FERMENTER'S NOTES

Produce: With some ferments, you can utilize produce that is slightly on the other side of fresh, but not with fruit ferments. You'll want to select the freshest fruit possible with no bruises or moldy spots. Overly ripe fruit can result in the formation of alcohol or a soft and mushy texture that's less than desirable.

Water: Good-quality spring or well water is ideal for the brined fruits in this section because it's full of minerals that the bacteria like. The fruit you'll be brining also contain plenty of these nutrients, so filtered or distilled water also works just fine.

Culture: Most of the recipes in this section call for a combination of salt (between 1.5 and 2%) and either kraut brine or whey as a starter culture. Keep in mind that more salt and starter up front means a longer shelf life in the refrigerator, but if you know you're going to eat the fruit within a week, you can slightly reduce both salt and starter.

Fermenting: Because fruit is so irresistible to yeasts and molds, it's even more important than with other ferments to keep the fruit fully submerged in the brine during and after fermentation. Use a weight or specialized fermentation disk (see page 49) to accomplish this. For jams and relishes, we have had good results laying a piece of cheesecloth, parchment paper, or plastic wrap in the jar on top of the ferment before sealing the jar.

Fermenting for just a day or two leaves a good amount of sugar in the fruit, and you'll hardly notice the difference. If you love sour like we do, go for a couple of days more. Five to seven days is the sweet spot for most of the fruit ferments in this chapter, but as you'll see the softer fruit are better suited to shorter fermentation times whereas firmer fruit such as apples can undergo longer fermentation times without it negatively affecting texture. The acidity of the lactic acid bacteria (LAB) enhances and brings out the full essence of the fruit's flavor while leaving behind just enough sugar for a slightly sweet finish.

Storage: If you think it may take you a while to get through your batch, we recommend transferring the fermented fruit into smaller containers. This tactic reduces the exposure to oxygen every time you open the jar as well as spoilage microbes that may try to sneak in on utensils or curious fingers. If, after a few weeks in the fridge, your ferment has become bubbly, worry not—it's still safe, but maybe not as pleasing, to eat. The bubbles are the result of either alcohol formation or trapped carbon dioxide created by the LAB munching on sugar; a quick whiff will usually tell you which has occurred. If it's the former, adding that alcoholic fruit jam to plain soda water makes a delightfully relaxing beverage.

BRINED APPLES
with Tarragon

MAKES 1 QUART

500 milliliters distilled or spring water

15 grams unrefined sea salt

200 grams thinly sliced Granny Smith apples (about 2 medium)

200 grams thinly sliced Honeycrisp apple (about 1 large)

2 to 4 sprigs tarragon

50 milliliters natural brine from Basic Kraut (page 92) or from store-bought plain kraut

EQUIPMENT

Kitchen scale

1-quart or 1-liter glass jar

Weight

Fermentation lid

The idea for this recipe was inspired by the Russian Brined Apples from Linda Ziedrich's *Joy of Pickling*. The traditional recipe called for whole yellow-skinned apples, along with honey and mint, but perhaps what we found most interesting about it was that a rye sourdough starter was used to start fermentation. Intrigued, we began to play around with different versions—and honestly, the sourdough thing just wasn't for us. We replaced it with kraut brine, and then swapped out the mint for tarragon, which took the ferment in very different direction and gave it a decidedly French feel. Rather than whole yellow apples, we found that a combination of Granny Smith and Honeycrisp slices accelerated fermentation time, and the firm flesh of these apple varieties stood up well to brining. We landed pretty far from the original, but we think the result is fantastic. The tarragon comes through nicely and complements the slightly sweet, salty, and tart flavors of the apples. This ferment pairs beautifully with cheeses, especially soft, pungent varieties like La Tur and Brie. Voilà!

Fermentation Temperature & Time

Above 68°F	Ferment 5 days or less
65° to 68°F	Ferment 6 days
Ideal: 64°F	Ferment 7 days
60° to 63°F	Ferment 8 to 9 days
Below 60°F	Ferment 10 days or more

1. Wash and sanitize all your fermentation equipment, including a knife and cutting board, and set aside to air-dry.

2. Make a salt brine by bringing 150 milliliters of the water to just under a boil in a small saucepan. Remove from the heat, add the salt, and stir well until all the salt has dissolved. Add the remaining 350 milliliters room-temperature water to the hot brine to cool it down; set aside.

3. Pack the apple slices into the jar and insert the sprigs of tarragon between the slices. Pour the kraut brine into the jar over the apples. Pour the salt brine into the jar, leaving about 2 inches of headspace. Reserve the extra salt brine in a small jar in the refrigerator to use as needed.

4. Place the weight in the jar on top of the apples and press down until the apples are completely submerged in the brine. Seal the jar with the fermentation lid. Place the sealed jar on a plate or in a bowl to catch any liquid displaced through the airlock during fermentation.

5. Ferment the apples in a cool place away from direct sunlight (7 days at 64°F is ideal—see the chart at left). Taste the apples after 5 days to determine if the flavor and sourness are to your liking. If they're not sour enough, reseal the jar and let them ferment for 2 days, then taste again. When the apples are to your liking, replace the fermentation lid with a regular lid, seal, and store in the refrigerator for up to 1 month.

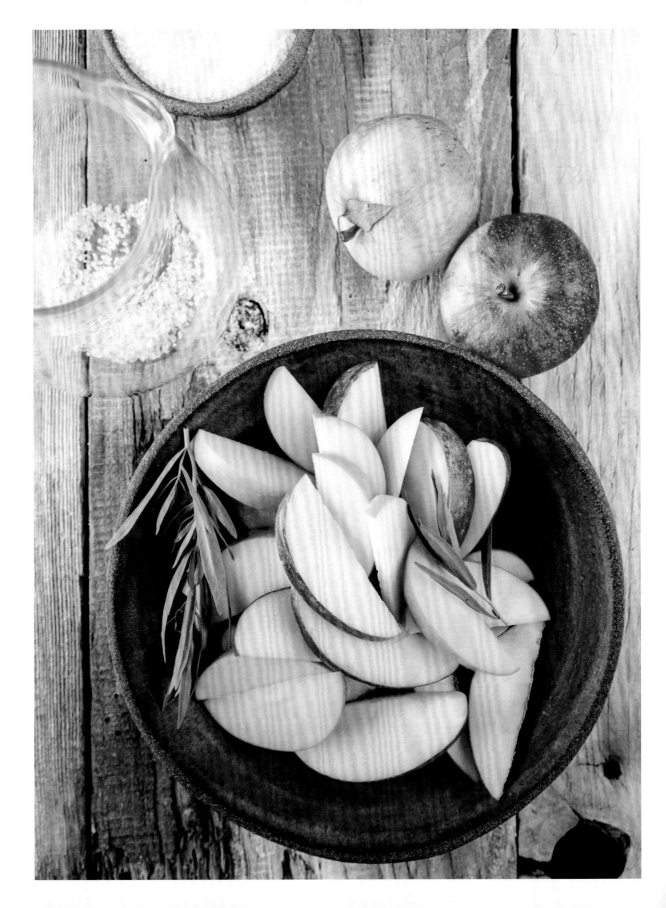

960 milliliters distilled or spring water

40 grams unrefined sea salt

860 grams sliced peeled watermelon rinds (1-inch-wide by 4- to 6-inch-long strips; see Notes)

30 grams thinly sliced peeled fresh ginger (from one roughly 4-inch piece)

30 grams coarsely chopped candied ginger

10 grams fresh Makrut lime leaves (about 10)

¼ teaspoon red pepper flakes

100 milliliters natural brine from Basic Kraut (page 92) or from store-bought plain kraut

EQUIPMENT

Kitchen scale

½-gallon or 2-liter glass jar

Weight (optional)

Fermentation lid

SPICY GINGER–MAKRUT LIME WATERMELON RINDS

About 40 percent of the weight of a watermelon is in the rind, so rather than tossing it, why not make a scrumptious pickle? Most of the work is in the peeling, but that goes quickly once you find your rhythm. We prefer slicing the rinds into spears so they're easy to grab from the jar, but you can cut them any way you like. The rinds have a tendency to float, so make sure to weight them down so they stay submerged in the brine. Fresh Makrut lime leaves are so much better than dried; they're typically available at natural foods stores and gourmet grocers, but if you can't find them, substitute sliced lime in the same quantity.

The fermented rinds are fabulous chopped and added to a salad, or you can do as we do in our house and eat them straight out of the jar like a dill pickle.

1. Wash and sanitize all your fermentation equipment, including a knife and cutting board, and set aside to air-dry.

2. Make a salt brine by bringing 300 milliliters of the water to just under a boil in a small saucepan. Remove from the heat, add the salt, and stir well until all the salt has dissolved. Add the remaining 660 milliliters room-temperature water to the hot brine to cool it down; set aside.

3. Put the watermelon rinds in the jar, packing them in upright, adding both types of ginger, the lime leaves, and the red pepper flakes as you go. Pour the kraut brine into the jar over the rinds. Pour the salt brine into the jar, leaving about 2 inches of headspace. Reserve the extra salt brine in a small jar in the refrigerator to use as needed.

4. Place the weight in the jar on top of the rinds and press down until the rinds are completely submerged in the brine (see Notes). Seal the jar with the fermentation lid. Place the sealed jar on a plate or in a bowl to catch any liquid displaced through the airlock during fermentation.

5. Ferment the rinds in a cool place away from direct sunlight (7 days at 64°F is ideal—see the chart on page 260). Taste the rinds after 5 days to determine if the flavor and sourness are to your liking (remember to use a clean utensil and never double dip). If they're not sour enough, reseal the jar and let them ferment for another day or two, then taste again. When the rinds are to your liking, replace the fermentation lid with a regular lid, seal, and store in the refrigerator for up to 3 months.

Notes: To prep the watermelon rinds, set a large bowl on your scale and tare the scale. Cut a whole watermelon into quarters or eighths. Remove the pink flesh from the rinds and reserve the flesh for another use. Using a sharp paring knife, peel the green skin from the rinds; discard the skin. Cut the rinds into 1-inch-thick, 4- to 6-inch long strips (or into chunks or any other shape you like), adding them to the bowl as you go until you have 860 grams.

Instead of using a specialized fermentation disk or weight, cut a rind into a round that fits into the top of the jar and use it to keep the other rinds submerged in the brine.

BRINED GINGER BLUEBERRIES

480 milliliters distilled or spring water

20 grams unrefined sea salt

400 grams fresh blueberries (a little more than a pint)

25 grams chopped candied ginger

10 grams grated peeled fresh ginger (from one roughly 2-inch piece)

50 milliliters natural brine from Basic Kraut (page 92) or from store-bought plain kraut

EQUIPMENT

Kitchen scale

1-quart or 1-liter wide-mouth glass jar

Canning funnel (optional)

Weight

Fermentation lid

The first time I tasted pickled blueberries a few years ago in Oregon, I nearly fainted with joy. It had never crossed my mind to douse berries with vinegar, but the combination, served on a goat cheese crostini, was spectacular. Shane and I began experimenting and came up with this lacto-fermented version. They are great in a salad (use the brine for the dressing), and equally so on yogurt with a drizzle of honey.

Both frozen and fresh berries work, but fresh keep their shape better and are our preference. Make sure to finely grate the ginger so the flavor can penetrate the berries. The candied ginger serves to balance the sweet and the sour in the ferment, so if you're going for full-on sour, replace it with the same amount of grated fresh ginger. —Kathryn

1. Wash and sanitize all your fermentation equipment, including a large bowl, knife, and cutting board, and set aside to air-dry.

2. Make a salt brine by bringing 145 milliliters of the water to just under a boil in a small saucepan. Remove from the heat, add the salt, and stir well until all the salt has dissolved. Add the remaining 335 milliliters room-temperature water to the hot brine to cool it down; set aside.

3. Lightly rinse the berries and transfer to the large bowl. Add both types of ginger. Using your hands, mix the berries and ginger until well combined. Transfer the berry mixture to the jar (a canning funnel is helpful here). Pour the kraut brine into the jar over the berry mixture. Pour the salt brine into the jar, leaving about 2 inches of headspace. Reserve the extra salt brine in a small jar in the refrigerator to use as needed.

4. Place the weight in the jar on top of the berry mixture and press down until the berry mixture is completely submerged in the brine. Seal the jar with the fermentation lid. Place the sealed jar on a plate or in a bowl to catch any liquid displaced through the airlock during fermentation.

5. Ferment the berry mixture in a cool place away from direct sunlight (7 days at 64°F is ideal—see the chart on page 260). Taste the berries after 5 days to determine if the flavor and sourness are to your liking (remember to use a clean utensil and never double dip). If they're not sour enough, reseal the jar and let them ferment for another 1 to 2 days, then taste again. When the berries are to your liking, replace the fermentation lid with a regular lid, seal, and store in the refrigerator for up to 1 month.

RASPBERRY-CHIA JAM

MAKES 1 PINT

445 grams fresh raspberries

25 grams chia seeds

5 grams unrefined sea salt

1 teaspoon good-quality pure vanilla extract

25 milliliters whey (see Note, page 271) or natural brine from Basic Kraut (page 92)

EQUIPMENT

Kitchen scale

Food processor

1-pint or ½-liter wide-mouth glass jar

Parchment paper or cheesecloth cut to the diameter of the jar

Fermentation lid

Sarah Wilson of *I Quit Sugar* fame is a woman fiercely committed to living an authentic life, and her cookbook is genius. Instead of making jam with loads of sugar and added pectin, she uses chia seeds (which are high in omega-3s and a great source of fiber) to gel the mixture, resulting in a firm, spreadable jam. Like we said, genius.

We prefer whey as a starter in this recipe, but if you're fresh out, kraut brine works well, although it will make the jam a little more tart. And in case you're wondering, the small amount of salt in the recipe is there to reduce the possibility of alcohol fermentation. Depending on how ripe the berries are, you may find yourself wanting to add a little sweetener. Because this a short ferment, you can sweeten it up front or as you use the jam. This second option allows you to use the jam in both sweet and savory dishes, which we find pretty appealing. In keeping with the "low-sugar spirit" of this recipe, we recommend a low-glycemic sweetener like brown rice syrup, coconut sugar, or, if you can tolerate it, stevia. With that said, you can't beat a good local honey. Thank you, Sarah, for inspiring this lacto-fermented jam!

1. Wash and sanitize all your fermentation equipment, including a medium bowl, knife, and cutting board, and set aside to air-dry.

2. In the food processor, combine the raspberries, chia seeds, salt, and vanilla and process until a thick paste forms. Transfer the raspberry mixture to the medium bowl, add the whey or kraut brine, and gently stir to combine.

3. Transfer the raspberry mixture to the jar, leaving about 1 inch of headspace. Place the parchment paper or cheesecloth in the jar over the raspberry mixture (the mixture should be completely covered). Seal the jar with the fermentation lid. Place the sealed jar on a plate or in a bowl to catch any liquid displaced through the airlock during fermentation.

4. Ferment the raspberry mixture in a cool place away from direct sunlight (2 days at 64°F is ideal—see the chart at right). Taste the jam after 2 days to determine if the flavor and sourness are to your liking (remember to use a clean utensil and never double dip). If it's not sour enough, reseal the jar and let it ferment for another day, then taste again. When the jam is to your liking, replace the fermentation lid with a regular lid, seal, and store in the refrigerator for up to 2 months.

Fermentation Temperature & Time

Above 68°F
Ferment 1 day

65° to 68°F
Ferment 1 to 2 days

Ideal: 64°F
Ferment 2 days

60° to 63°F
Ferment 2 to 3 days

Below 60°F
Ferment 3 days

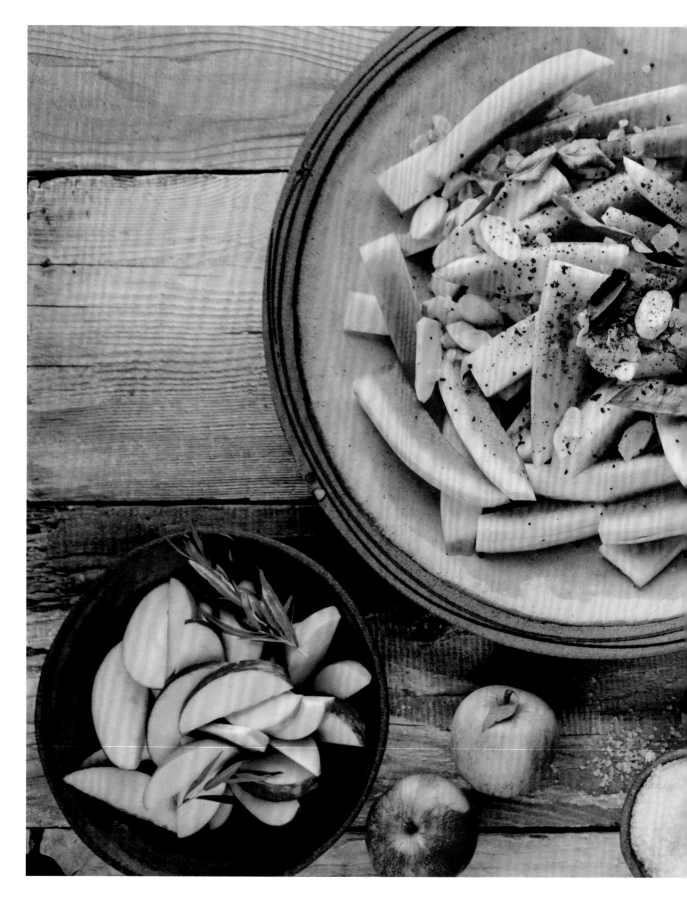

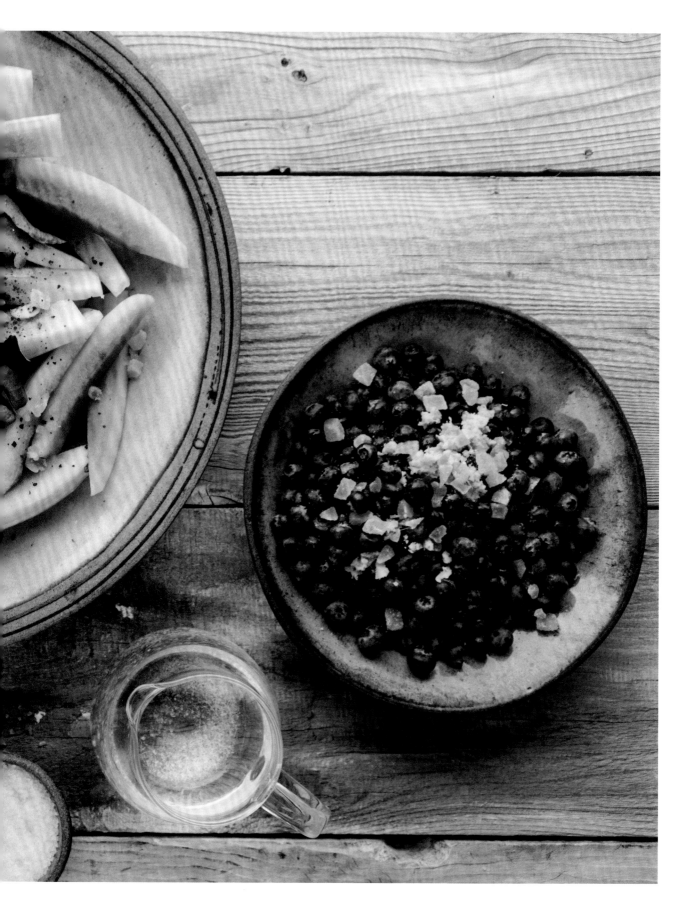

200 grams sliced Granny Smith apples (about 2 medium; sliced into eighths)

510 grams fresh or thawed frozen cranberries

100 grams walnuts or other nut of your choice

2 teaspoons lemon zest

30 milliliters lemon juice (from about 1 lemon)

1 tablespoon orange zest

75 milliliters fresh orange juice (from about 1 orange)

2 teaspoons ground cinnamon

¼ teaspoon ground cloves

20 grams unrefined sea salt

50 milliliters natural brine from Basic Kraut (page 92) or whey (see Note, page 271)

EQUIPMENT

Kitchen scale

Food processor

1-quart or 1-liter glass jar

Parchment paper or cheesecloth cut to the diameter of the jar

Fermentation lid

CRANBERRY-ORANGE-WALNUT RELISH

Most of us think of cranberries as a holiday treat, but we ask you to consider eating them on a regular basis for their amazing health benefits. Ladies know how effective pure cranberry juice (not the sugary stuff) can be for preventing and treating urinary tract infections, but did you know that this little berry has one of the highest concentrations of antioxidants of any fruit? They are anti-inflammatory, immune boosting, and may help prevent cancer and reduce the risk of heart disease. Recent research has shown that cranberries also help optimize the balance of bacteria in our guts. And finally, they're diuretic, so they help with detoxification and water retention. Great, right? The problem is that you need to eat them raw in order to get most of these health benefits, and their tartness and astringency are just a little too intense for most of us. Fermentation to the rescue! After a few days in the crock, these berries mellow considerably but retain all their superpowers. And, of course, you've invited a big dose of live cultures to the party.

Both fresh and frozen cranberries work beautifully in this relish; if using frozen, just thaw them before starting. We use walnuts because they're our local nut, but pecans, hazelnuts, or even almonds would also be excellent choices. (You could also leave them out altogether and replace the loss of volume with an equal weight of cranberries or even apples.)

Although substantially subdued by fermentation, this relish is still tart. It's fantastic with goat cheese or yogurt, whirled into a smoothie, or scattered over a salad. And if you want it sweeter, add a wee bit of honey or your favorite sweetener right before eating. For the holidays, use this as the base for a cranberry sauce, adding water and Cointreau or Grand Marnier, cooking it down for 10 minutes, and finishing it, off the heat, with a little orange zest and honey. Cheers!

1. Wash and sanitize all your fermentation equipment, including a large bowl, knife, and cutting board, and set aside to air-dry.

2. In a food processor, pulse the apples until broken down to about the size of the cranberries. Add the cranberries, walnuts, lemon zest, lemon juice, orange zest, orange juice, cinnamon, cloves, and salt to the processor bowl and pulse until the mixture is coarsely chopped. Transfer the relish to a large bowl and gently stir in the kraut brine or whey.

3. Transfer the relish to the jar, leaving about 1 inch of headspace. Place the parchment paper or cheesecloth in the jar over the relish (the relish should be completely covered). Seal the jar with the fermentation lid. Place the jar on a plate or in a bowl to catch any liquid displaced through the airlock during fermentation.

4. Ferment the relish in a cool place away from direct sunlight (5 days at 64°F is ideal—see the chart at right). Taste the relish after 3 days to determine if the flavor and sourness are to your liking (remember to use a clean utensil and never double dip). If it's not sour enough, reseal the jar and let it ferment for another day or two, then taste again. When the relish is to your liking, replace the fermentation lid with a regular lid, seal, and store in the refrigerator for up to 3 months.

Fermentation Temperature & Time

Above 68°F
Ferment 3 days or less

65° to 68°F
Ferment 4 days

Ideal: 64°F
Ferment 5 days

60° to 63°F
Ferment 6 days

Below 60°F
Ferment 7 days or more

---

200 milliliters distilled or spring water

5 grams unrefined sea salt

450 grams sliced fresh peaches (sliced into eighths)

220 milliliters fresh vanilla whey (see Note), at room temperature

½ teaspoon good-quality pure vanilla extract

EQUIPMENT

Kitchen scale

1-quart or 1-liter glass jar

Weight

Fermentation lid

Fermentation Temperature & Time

Above 68°F
Ferment 1 day

65° to 68°F
Ferment 1 to 2 days

Ideal: 64°F
Ferment 2 days

60° to 63°F
Ferment 2 to 3 days

Below 60°F
Ferment 3 days

VANILLA-WHEY PEACHES

This recipe is the result of a happy accident. I had picked up some yogurt at the grocery store for making yogurt cheese and whey, and it wasn't until I was done draining it that I discovered it was vanilla instead of plain. The whey was so incredibly delicious, I knew I had to make a fruit ferment with it, and peaches were calling me. Fond memories of hot summer afternoons when my grandfather would enlist all the kids to help him crank and churn vanilla custard into a creamy ice cream so we could top it with his luscious canned homegrown peaches sparked the idea for this recipe.

This recipe works best with fresh peaches. You'll love these whey peaches on yogurt or ice cream with a sprinkle of cinnamon, but you could also puree them with a little bourbon and honey to make a sweet-and-sour glaze for vegetables and meats. They complement mild, spreadable goat's- or sheep's-milk cheeses (or even yogurt cheese!) and are great on toast or crackers, topped with a little fresh basil or tarragon. Or just mix them into your fruit salad for a tangy, probiotic boost. Use the leftover whey on cereal or give your smoothie a dose of flavorful live cultures. Thank you, Grandpa John! —Kathryn

1. Wash and sanitize all your fermentation equipment, including a medium bowl, knife, and cutting board, and set aside to air-dry.

2. Make a brine by bringing 100 milliliters of the water to just under a boil in a small saucepan. Remove from the heat, add the salt, and stir well until all the salt has dissolved. Add the remaining 100 milliliters room-temperature water to the hot brine to cool it down; set aside.

3. In the medium bowl, combine the peaches, whey, and vanilla. Using your hands, gently mix to combine. Transfer the peaches along with any liquid to the jar. Pour the brine into the jar, leaving about 2 inches of headspace. Reserve the extra brine in a small jar in the refrigerator to use as needed.

4. Place the weight in the jar and press down until the peaches are completely submerged in the brine. Seal the jar with the fermentation lid. Place the sealed jar on a plate or in a bowl to catch any liquid displaced through the airlock during fermentation.

5. Ferment the peaches in a cool place away from direct sunlight (2 days at 64°F is ideal—see the chart opposite). Taste the peaches after 1 day to determine if the flavor and sourness are to your liking (remember to use a clean utensil and never double dip). If they're not sour enough, reseal the jar and let them ferment for another day or two, then taste again.

6. When the peaches are to your liking, replace the fermentation lid with a regular lid, seal, and store in the refrigerator for up to one week.

Note: To gather the whey for this recipe, start with 908 grams (2 pounds) of vanilla yogurt (whole milk, low fat, or nonfat). Make sure there are no preservatives or thickeners in the ingredient list and avoid using Greek yogurt—it's been strained already. Line a large strainer with cheesecloth or a thin, clean dish towel and set the strainer in a larger bowl. Pour the yogurt into the strainer, cover, and place in the refrigerator or on your counter for at least 4 hours or up to overnight. The whey will drain into the bowl, while the milk solids remain in the cloth. Reserve the strained yogurt for another use. Depending on the type of yogurt you've used, this should yield 300 to 400 milliliters of whey.

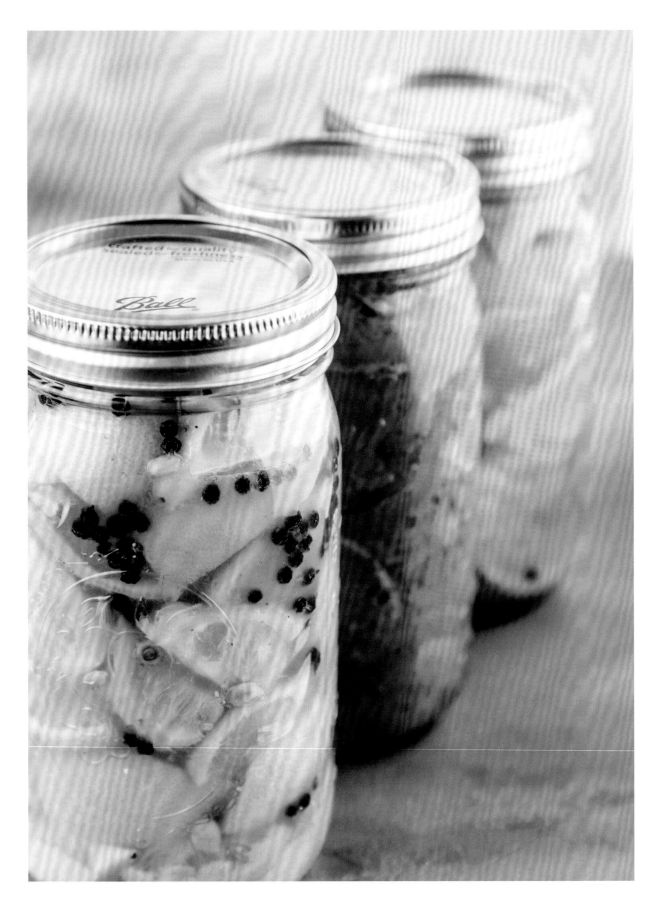

Preserved Citrus

Although we foodies tend to think of preserved lemons as Moroccan, historians speculate that this robust preserve may have originated in India, which would explain why they were so popular in eighteenth-century England. Limes pickled (brined) in seawater were imported by the barrel from the West Indies to North America throughout the nineteenth century, and those mouth-puckering treats were treasured by children in early American culture. Louisa May Alcott captured the zeitgeist in *Little Women* in this passage where twelve-year-old Amy attempts to explain the social importance of sour limes to her sisters Jo and Meg:

> Why, you see, the girls are always buying them, and unless you want to be thought mean, you must do it, too. It's nothing but limes now, for everyone is sucking them in their desks in school time, and trading them off for pencils, bead rings, paper dolls, or something else. . . . If one girl likes another, she gives her a lime; if she's mad with her, she eats one before her face, and doesn't offer even a suck. They treat by turns, and I've had ever so many but haven't returned them, and I ought, for they are debts of honor, you know.

We're not sure why pickled limes didn't survive into the twenty-first century, but we think they deserve to make a comeback. Wouldn't we rather our kids suck on salty sour limes and lemons full of vitamin C and beneficial live microbes than on artificially flavored sour candies?

But kids and their sugar consumption aside, preserved citrus is a decidedly grown-up ingredient. We use preserved citrus in small amounts to add concentrated citrus flavor, umami, and depth to so many dishes, it's hard to know where to start. It adds interest and depth to many pasta dishes—in fact, the first time I encountered preserved lemon was in an incredibly tasty crab risotto. Preserved lemons are used in numerous Middle Eastern dishes, but perhaps our favorite is Moroccan *djej makalli*, chicken stewed with olives and preserved lemons. In Vietnam, pickled lime juice is mixed with sweetener for a refreshing summer drink or a fortifying hot drink. No salad in our house is eaten without a little preserved lemon, lime, or orange either tossed into the salad or blended into the dressing. When you reach for a fresh lemon, ask yourself if a preserved one could take its place. We think you might soon find preserved citrus as indispensable as we do.

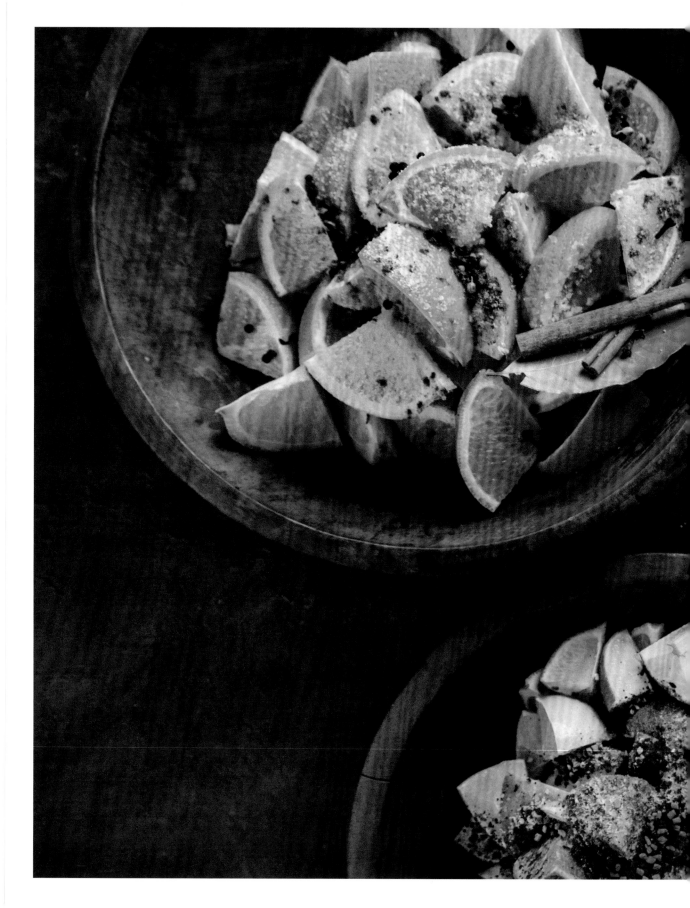

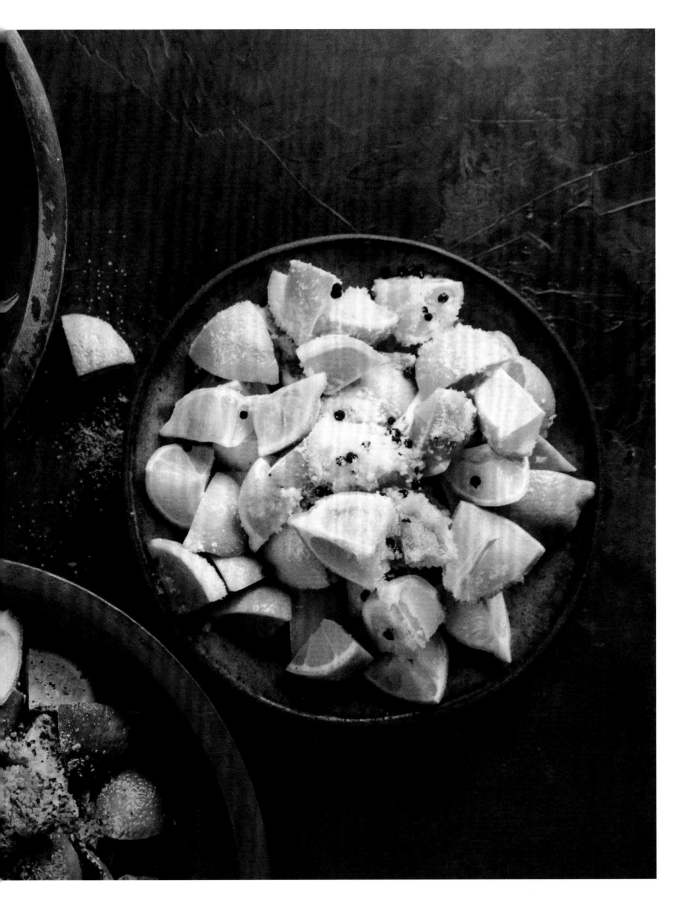

PRESERVED LEMONS
with Peppercorns

810 grams unwaxed lemons (preferably Meyer; about 8)

50 grams coarse unrefined sea salt, plus ½ teaspoon for sprinkling on top

15 grams whole black peppercorns

75 milliliters fresh lemon juice (from 2 to 3 lemons)

EQUIPMENT

Kitchen scale

1-quart or 1-liter wide-mouth glass jar

Canning funnel (optional)

Kraut tamper (optional)

Fermentation lid

The simplest preserved citrus recipe, these lemons can be made in a snap and, as mentioned on page 273, are a highly versatile ingredient with any number of culinary uses.

Although we've provided approximate quantities for how many lemons you'll need, keep in mind that these are averages. Meyer lemons yield quite a bit more juice than Eurekas, for instance, and seasonal variations can also affect juice quantity. If you stick to the weights given in the ingredients list, you should have just the right amount to fill your jar.

1. Wash and sanitize all your fermentation equipment, including a large bowl, knife, and cutting board, and set aside to air-dry. Set a large bowl on your scale and tare.

2. Thoroughly wash the lemons. Quarter them lengthwise, then slice each quarter in half crosswise (you should have 8 sections per lemon), adding them to the large bowl and weighing as you go.

3. Add the 50 grams salt and the peppercorns to the bowl with the lemons. Using your hands, lightly mix the lemon pieces with the salt and pepper until the lemons are well coated.

4. Transfer the lemons to the jar (a canning funnel is useful here and helps to minimize spillage). As you add them, tamp them down with your fist or a kraut tamper to expel some of their juice, submerge them under the natural brine that forms, and force out any air pockets. Continue until the jar is almost full, and then pour the 75 milliliters lemon juice over the lemons to cover, leaving 1 inch of headspace. Sprinkle the remaining ½ teaspoon salt evenly over the top of the lemons.

5. Seal the jar with the fermentation lid. Place the jar on a plate or in a bowl to catch any liquid displaced through the airlock during fermentation.

6. Ferment the lemons on your counter (5 weeks at 64°F is ideal—see the chart opposite). Test a piece lemon after 4 weeks to see if the rind has softened. If it's still tough, leave to ferment for another week and test again. Once the texture is to your liking, place the lemons in the refrigerator where they will last for up to one year.

7. To use, remove a lemon section from the jar and rinse it. Scrape out the pulp (discard it or use it to flavor dressings and sauces). Cut the rind into small dice or thin strips and add to your dish.

Variations

To make these variations, follow the same instructions as in the master formula, adding all the extra seasonings at the same time as the 50 grams of salt.

Spicy Indian Limes
MAKES 1 QUART

810 grams limes (10 to 12)

50 grams unrefined sea salt, plus 1 teaspoon for sprinkling

15 grams chili powder

7 grams ground turmeric

15 grams asafoetida

5 grams ground fenugreek seeds

75 milliliters fresh lime juice (from about 4 limes)

Moroccan Oranges
MAKES 1 QUART

810 grams oranges (5 to 7 medium)

50 grams unrefined sea salt, plus 1 teaspoon for sprinkling

15 grams whole black peppercorns

2 cinnamon sticks

½ teaspoon coriander seeds

½ teaspoon whole cloves

½ teaspoon ground allspice

1 bay leaf

75 milliliters fresh orange juice (from about 1 orange)

Fermentation Temperature & Time

Above 68°F
Ferment 4 weeks or less

65° to 68°F
Ferment 4 to 5 weeks

Ideal: 64°F
Ferment 5 weeks

60° to 63°F
Ferment 5 to 6 weeks

Below 60°F
Ferment 6 weeks or more

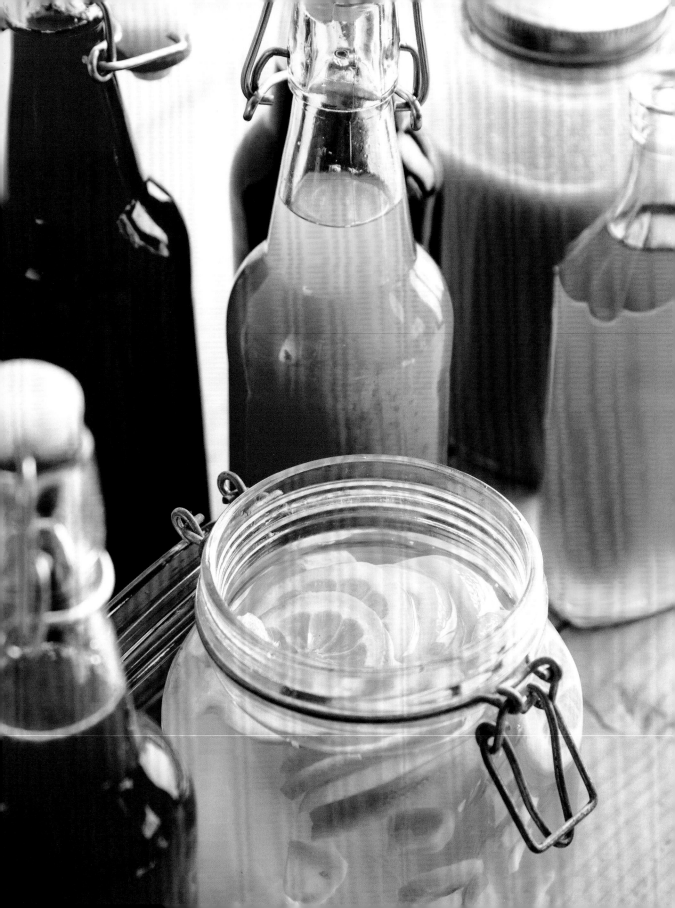

CHAPTER TEN

Sour Tonic (Kvass), Kombucha, and Water Kefir

In this chapter we will share with you our knowledge and passion for making live-cultured, nonalcoholic (or close to nonalcoholic) beverages. Sour tonics, kombucha, and water kefir are all wide ranging and unique ferments, but they do have some commonalities: they are all alive, tart, and delicious! All the following beverages could be considered healthy substitutes for sugar-laced soft drinks, and are pleasingly tart due to the acids produced through the fermentation.

Sour Tonics

Many cultures have their version of a salty sour tonic, typically consumed to aid digestion. These sour tonics are made from vegetables, such as beets, that are lacto-fermented in a low-salt brine (fruits are used less often). The other defining feature of this category of ferments is that the vegetables are fermented with a higher proportion of brine; with typical brined ferments you ferment at a ratio somewhere near 50/50 brine to solids, whereas sour tonics are fermented closer to a ratio of 75/25 brine to solids. In addition to the beet sour (also called beet kvass or beet *rassol*), one of the most common sour tonics, you can make sour tonics using any number of vegetables and fruits. In Eastern Europe and Russia, beets are king. In India, carrots form the base for the sour tonic *kaanji*. We have taken liberty with the traditional sour tonic recipe by adding fruits and spices to vegetable bases to create what we think are exciting flavor combinations. And because our sour tonics are lower in salt, we find them more refreshing.

Sour tonics are incredibly easy to make at home, offering many of the probiotic benefits of kombucha with none of the fuss or hassle of maintaining a SCOBY. Traditionally, sour tonic recipes do not include a secondary fermentation, but we find the resulting carbonation quite pleasing.

Carbonation also makes these beverages more closely resemble soda, albeit a much healthier version. Served still, carbonated, or lightly sweetened and flavored with fruit and spices, these sour tonics can form the base for a number of delicious drinks. Who knows—you might even be able to convince your kids to make the switch to this far-healthier alternative to juice or soda.

FERMENTER'S NOTES

Produce: To peel or not to peel? Mostly there is no need to peel, but it really depends on the vegetable or fruit and whether you plan to use the strained solids post-fermentation. In some cases, as with beets, we recommend peeling because you can use the fermented beets in a number of recipes, and they are much more appetizing without their skins.

Traditionally, leftover beet solids are used to make a wonderfully nourishing soup called borscht. You can also toss them into salads or salad dressings, and we've even found that they can be quite good blended into hummus—just make sure to eat the hummus within 2 to 3 days so the microbes don't start fermenting the hummus. To preserve fermented beets for later use, transfer them to a smaller jar, submerge them in fresh brine, and refrigerate for up to 2 months. To make fresh brine, combine 15 grams unrefined salt with 485 milliliters distilled or spring water (500 milliliters of brine should be plenty). One of our favorite ways to use the leftover fermented beets is to turn them into fruit leather. All the recipes in this section can be transformed into delicious fruit leathers, except the Kaanji and the Lime-Mint Cucumber Sour, neither of which we recommend. To make fruit leather, simply combine the leftover vegetable/fruit solids in a blender with 2 to 3 tablespoons honey, and blend until you achieve a smooth puree. The honey helps to cut some of the sourness of the fermented vegetables, but you can omit the honey if you are weary of sugar. If your blender is sticking, you can add a small portion (50 milliliters or so) of your sour tonic to the mix in order to assist the blending process. Spread the puree in a thin, even layer (about ⅛ inch thick) on dehydrator sheets or a baking sheet lined with parchment paper, and dehydrate until the puree is firm but still slightly sticky to the touch (about 4 hours at 150°F in a dehydrator, or on the lowest setting of your oven for a much shorter period (1 to 2 hours), keeping a vigilant eye on it so as not to over-crisp). Peel the veggie/fruit leather off the sheet, cut into strips, and store in an airtight container for up to 6 months.

Some folks reuse the vegetables to make a second batch of tonic, but we generally don't recommend this; the vegetables have a tendency to get "funky" during the second fermentation, and we've consistently encountered issues with yeast and/or mold. The second batch is also less flavorful. If fruit is mixed in with the vegetables, you absolutely *cannot* use them second time.

Water: Good-quality spring or well water is ideal for making sour tonics because it's full of minerals that the bacteria like. The vegetables and fruit you'll be fermenting also contain plenty of these nutrients, though, so filtered or distilled water works just fine.

Brine: These sour tonic recipes are designed to make extra brine, which should be reserved and stored in the refrigerator, where it will keep for seven to ten days. This brine can be used if you lose some of the brine through the airlock or lid during the fermentation process. If this happens, open the jar, add the replacement brine, leaving 2 inches of headspace, and reseal (leave the jar open only as long as it takes to add the brine, to avoid introducing unwanted yeasts and molds). During the first five to seven days, gas (CO_2) is produced, which can cause the brine to be expelled through the airlock, potentially dropping the brine level below the vegetables. If you add replacement brine too soon, it will just be expelled by the gases, too, so wait until the end of this first phase before adding more brine. The exposed vegetables are protected by a layer of CO_2 during this phase and generally will not deteriorate. You'll know this phase is complete when the brine stops bubbling.

Culture: Because our sour tonics are relatively low in salt, it's imperative to use a starter culture. We use our Basic Kraut brine (page 92) as the starter culture in our sour tonic recipes, but you can also use other starter cultures (see page 64 for more on starter cultures).

Fermenting: Because of the tonics' lower salt content, we advise fermenting at or below 64°F, in order to give the lactic acid bacteria (LAB) an edge over yeasts and molds. If you know your fermentation temperature will be above 68°F, it might be a good idea to increase the salt incrementally, depending on the temperature. Fruit can also be a source of yeast, and sometimes mold, which can result in off flavors and higher alcohol production. Usually a thorough scrubbing will do, but if you suspect mold or yeast is present on your fruit, soak the fruit in distilled white vinegar for 10 minutes and then rinse with fresh water before starting your sour tonic. Using the freshest ingredients available can also make a difference to the success of your sour tonic.

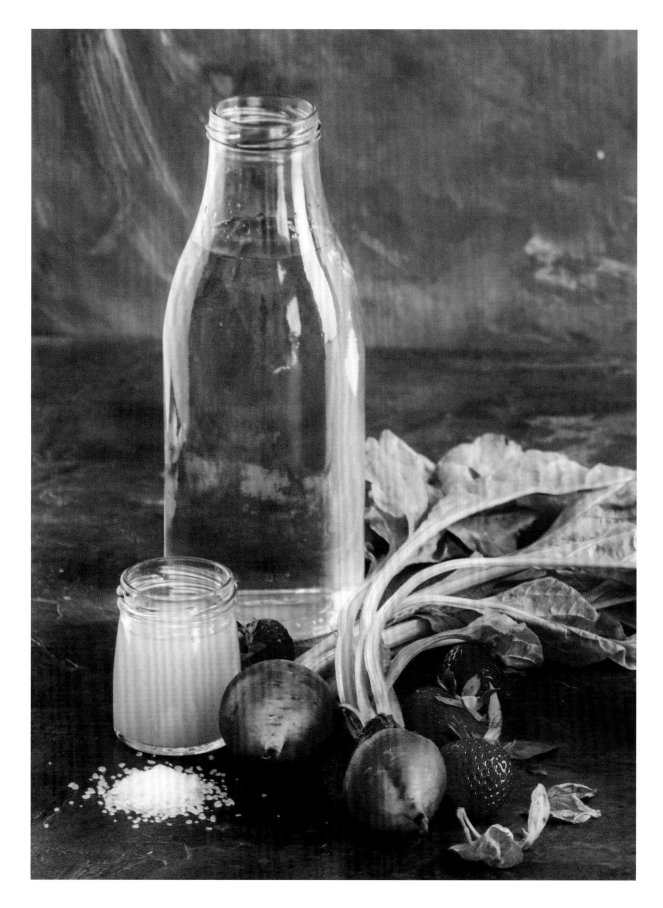

STRAWBERRY-BASIL BEET SOUR

MAKES ½ GALLON

1,490 milliliters distilled or spring water

10 grams unrefined sea salt

250 grams diced peeled red beets (½-inch cubes)

145 grams destemmed fresh whole strawberries, lightly muddled

5 grams fresh basil leaves

100 milliliters natural brine from Basic Kraut (page 92) or 100 grams Basic Kraut

EQUIPMENT

Kitchen scale

½-gallon or 2-liter wide-mouth glass jar

Fermentation lid

3 (16-ounce) flip-top bottles

Beet sour, also commonly referred to as beet kvass or *rassol* (Russian for "brine"), is a beautiful and healing lacto-fermented sour tonic with origins in Ukraine and Eastern Europe, where it has been consumed for at least a thousand years. The word *kvass* broadly refers to a variety of fermented drinks, the most common of which is made with dark bread fermented with yeast, and as a result is slightly alcoholic and resembles a beer more than a sour tonic. More aptly named beet sour, this lacto-fermented sour beverage is considered an excellent blood tonic, digestive aid, and liver cleanser. Beets are naturally high in phytonutrients called betalains, which are both antioxidant and anti-inflammatory. Beets naturally contain nitrates, but the fermentation process converts nitrates to nitric oxide, which increases blood flow to the brain and improves cognitive function. With this sour tonic, you reap all the health benefits beets have to offer, with the added benefit that the fermentation process makes their nutrients more bioavailable.

This was one of the first beet sours we ever made, and it's still a favorite. Both fresh and frozen strawberries work beautifully, but make sure to thaw the frozen berries before starting. Basil is a nice subtle accompaniment to the fruitiness of the strawberries, the earthiness of the beets, and the tanginess that results from the fermentation. For secondary fermentation, use a combination of fresh and freeze-dried strawberries for a truly delightful bubbly brew.

1. Wash and sanitize all your fermentation equipment, including a knife and cutting board, and set aside to air-dry.

2. Make a salt brine by bringing 300 milliliters of the water to just under a boil in a small saucepan. Remove from the heat, add the salt, and stir well until all the salt has dissolved. Add the remaining 1,190 milliliters room-temperature water to the hot brine to cool it down; set aside.

3. Combine the beets, strawberries, and basil in the jar. Pour the kraut brine into the jar over the beets and berries. Pour the salt brine into the jar, leaving about 2 inches of headspace. Reserve the extra salt brine in a small jar in the refrigerator to use as needed. Seal the jar with the fermentation lid. Place the jar on a plate or in a bowl to catch any liquid displaced through the airlock during fermentation.

4. Ferment the beet mixture in a cool place away from direct sunlight (2 weeks at 64°F is ideal—see the chart at right). Taste the beet mixture after 1 week to determine if the sourness is to your liking. If it's not sour enough, reseal the jar and leave it to ferment for another week, then taste again. When the beet mixture is sour to your liking, strain it through a fine-mesh sieve set over a bowl; discard the beets or reserve them for another use (see page 283). Transfer the liquid into bottles, seal, and store in the refrigerator for up to 6 months. Enjoy the beet sour still, or add flavoring and/or carbonation through a secondary fermentation in the bottle (see step 6 on page 329).

Fermentation Temperature & Time

Above 68°F
Ferment 1 week or less

65° to 68°F
Ferment 1 to 2 weeks

Ideal: 64°F
Ferment 2 weeks

60° to 63°F
Ferment 2 to 3 weeks

Below 60°F
Ferment 3 weeks or more

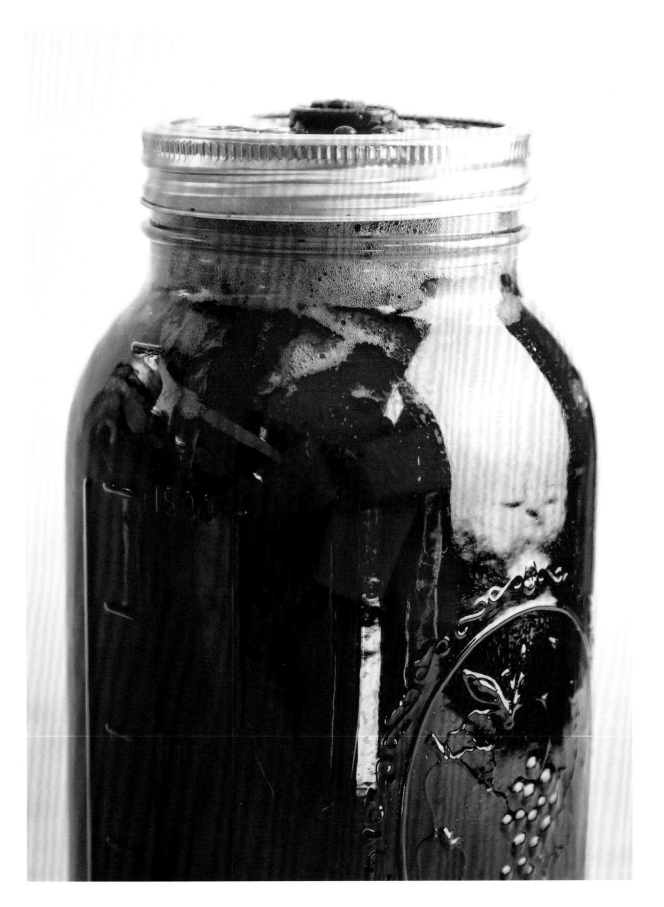

BLUEBERRY-GINGER BEET SOUR

MAKES ½ GALLON

1,490 milliliters distilled or spring water

10 grams unrefined sea salt

260 grams diced peeled red beets (½-inch cubes)

100 grams blueberries, muddled

40 grams coarsely chopped peeled fresh ginger

100 milliliters natural brine from Basic Kraut (page 92) or 100 grams Basic Kraut

EQUIPMENT

Kitchen scale

½-gallon or 2-liter wide-mouth glass jar

Fermentation lid

3 (16-ounce) flip-top bottles

The sweetness of blueberries and the spiciness of ginger beautifully complement the earthiness of the beets in this recipe. The sugars in the fruit also serve as another food source for the bacteria, and can slightly accelerate the fermentation time. A shorter fermentation time will allow more of the fruit flavors to come through, while a longer one will result in a more "sour" flavor profile. A secondary fermentation using additional fruit will reintroduce sweetness and flavor and create delightfully bubbly soda. You can also add some dried blueberries to the bottles to punch up the blueberry flavor during the secondary fermentation.

1. Wash and sanitize all your fermentation equipment, including a knife and cutting board, and set aside to air-dry.

2. Make a salt brine by bringing 300 milliliters of the water to just under a boil in a small saucepan. Remove from the heat, add the salt, and stir well until all the salt has dissolved. Add the remaining 1,190 milliliters room-temperature water to the hot brine to cool it down; set aside.

3. Combine the beets, blueberries, and ginger in the jar. Pour the kraut brine into the jar over the beets and blueberries. Pour the salt brine into the jar, leaving about 2 inches of headspace. Reserve the extra salt brine in a small jar in the refrigerator to use as needed. Seal the jar with the fermentation lid. Place the jar on a plate or in a bowl to catch any liquid displaced through the airlock during fermentation.

4. Ferment the beet mixture in a cool place away from direct sunlight (2 weeks at 64°F is ideal—see the chart on page 287). Taste the beet mixture after 1 week to determine if the sourness is to your liking. If it's not sour enough, reseal the jar and leave it to ferment for another week, then taste again.

5. When the beet mixture is sour to your liking, strain it through a fine-mesh sieve set over a bowl; discard the beets or reserve them for another use (see page 283). Transfer the liquid into bottles, seal, and store in the refrigerator for up to 6 months. Enjoy the beet sour still, or add flavoring and/or carbonation through a secondary fermentation in the bottle (see step 6 on page 329).

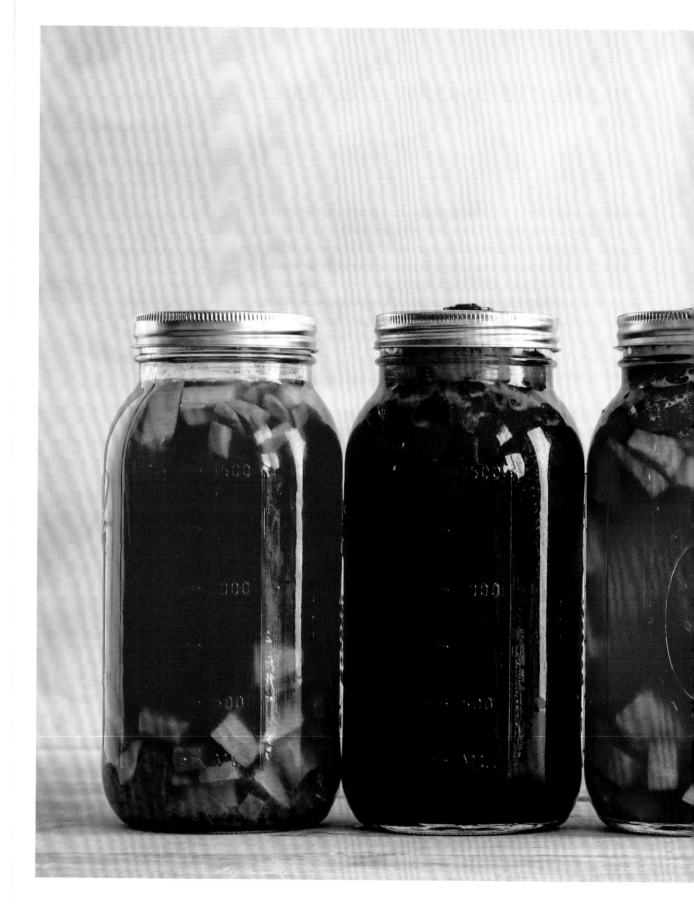

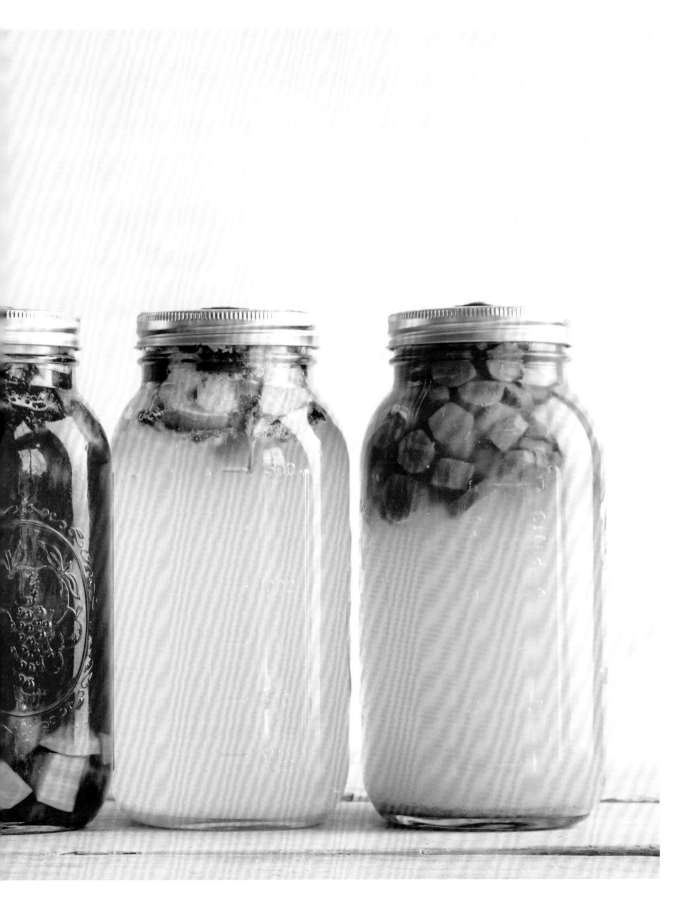

TANGERINE-TURMERIC BEET SOUR

1,440 milliliters distilled or spring water

10 grams unrefined sea salt

300 grams diced peeled golden beets (½-inch cubes)

50 grams grated peeled fresh turmeric (from about two 4-inch pieces)

1 tablespoon tangerine zest

100 milliliters tangerine juice (from 3 or 4 tangerines)

2 cinnamon sticks

1 teaspoon whole black peppercorns

100 milliliters natural brine from Basic Kraut (page 92) or 100 grams Basic Kraut

EQUIPMENT

Kitchen scale

½-gallon or 2-liter wide-mouth glass jar

Fermentation lid

3 (16-ounce) bottles

You might think adding acidity to something that's already sour is redundant, but in the case of citrus and sour tonics, this is not always true. In this recipe, for instance, the floral sweetness and gentle acidity of tangerine balance and mellow the stronger lactic acidity found in sour tonics. During secondary fermentation, we like to add a touch of tangerine juice and a couple of dried orange sections to revive some of the citrus notes lost during the initial fermentation.

Turmeric root adds gorgeous color, a tiny note of bitter, and amazing anti-inflammatory properties, making this a truly healing tonic.

1. Wash and sanitize all your fermentation equipment, including a knife and cutting board, and set aside to air-dry.

2. Make a salt brine by bringing 300 milliliters of the water to just under a boil in a small saucepan. Remove from the heat, add the salt, and stir well until all the salt has dissolved. Add the remaining 1,140 milliliters room-temperature water to the hot brine to cool it down; set aside.

3. Combine the beets, turmeric, tangerine zest, tangerine juice, cinnamon sticks, and peppercorns in the jar. Pour the kraut brine into the jar over the beets. Pour the salt brine into the jar, leaving about 2 inches of headspace. Reserve the extra salt brine in a small jar in the refrigerator to use as needed. Seal the jar with the fermentation lid. Place the jar on a plate or in a bowl to catch any liquid displaced through the airlock during fermentation.

4. Ferment the beet mixture in a cool place away from direct sunlight (2 weeks at 64°F is ideal—see the chart on page 287). Taste the beet mixture after 1 week to determine if the sourness is to your liking. If it's not sour enough, reseal the jar and leave it to ferment for another week, then taste again.

5. When the beet mixture is sour to your liking, strain it through a fine-mesh sieve set over a bowl; discard the beets or reserve them for another use (see page 283). Transfer the liquid into bottles, seal, and store in the refrigerator for up to 6 months. Enjoy the beet sour still, or add flavoring and/or carbonation through a secondary fermentation in the bottle (see step 6 on page 329).

GINGER-PEAR BEET SOUR

Whoever said pears get ten minutes of fame when fully ripe was so right! This sour tonic is just the right place for pear starlets to play their one last great role. There is a fine line between a slightly overripe pear and a rotten one, and unless you want to make hooch, it's important to avoid rotten. Fresh ginger loves pear, of course, and is all too happy to play a supporting role here. You can also substitute apples for the pears in this recipe for another tasty variation. For the finale, add candied ginger to the secondary fermentation to pick up where the fresh ginger left off and to create a burst of sweetness and bubbles.

MAKES ½ GALLON

1,490 milliliters distilled or spring water

10 grams unrefined sea salt

200 grams diced peeled golden beets (½-inch cubes)

160 grams coarsely chopped Bartlett or other soft-fleshed pears

40 grams grated peeled fresh ginger

100 milliliters natural brine from Basic Kraut (page 92) or 100 grams Basic Kraut

EQUIPMENT

Kitchen scale

½-gallon or 2-liter wide-mouth glass jar

Fermentation lid

3 (16-ounce) bottles

1. Wash and sanitize all your fermentation equipment, including a knife and cutting board, and set aside to air-dry.

2. Make a salt brine by bringing 300 milliliters of the water to just under a boil in a small saucepan. Remove from the heat, add the salt, and stir well until all the salt has dissolved. Add the remaining 1,190 milliliters room-temperature water to the hot brine to cool it down, set aside.

3. Combine the beets, pear, and ginger in the jar. Pour the kraut brine into the jar over the beets and pears. Pour the salt brine into the jar, leaving about 2 inches of headspace. Reserve the extra salt brine in a small jar in the refrigerator to use as needed. Seal the jar with the fermentation lid. Place the jar on a plate or in a bowl to catch any liquid displaced through the airlock during fermentation.

4. Ferment the beet mixture in a cool place away from direct sunlight (2 weeks at 64°F is ideal—see the chart on page 287). Taste the beet mixture after 1 week to determine if the sourness is to your liking. If it's not sour enough, reseal the jar and leave it to ferment for another week, then taste again.

5. When the beet mixture is sour to your liking, strain it through a fine-mesh sieve set over a bowl; discard the beets or reserve them for another use (see page 283). Transfer the liquid into bottles, seal, and store in the refrigerator for up to 6 months. Enjoy the beet sour still, or add flavoring and/or carbonation through a secondary fermentation in the bottle (see step 6 on page 329).

CARROT-LEMON SOUR

1,430 milliliters distilled or spring water

10 grams unrefined sea salt

400 grams sliced carrots (¼-inch-thick rounds)

1 tablespoon lemon zest

60 milliliters lemon juice (from 2 lemons)

½ to 1 teaspoons cayenne pepper

100 milliliters natural brine from Basic Kraut (page 92) or 100 grams Basic Kraut

EQUIPMENT

Kitchen scale

½-gallon or 2-liter wide-mouth glass jar

Fermentation lid

3 (16-ounce) bottles

The Master Cleanse consists of unlimited quantities of one drink—a concoction of water, lemon juice, maple syrup, and cayenne—and nothing else for ten days. Some find it controversial, but new research suggests that there might be a lot more to fasting than just shedding pounds. Not asking your body to digest food for a few days appears to give the gut lining a chance to heal and may help reset the balance of gut microbes. This recipe was inspired by the Master Cleanse, but with the addition of carrots and fermentation, it is something quite different altogether. Carrots and lemon are a perfect pairing, and the lemon serves to mask some of the off-flavors that you can get when fermenting carrots. We like the cayenne to be an accent flavor; at the lower end of suggested range, it adds just a touch of spice. If you really like heat and want to create a spicier version, you can opt for the greater quantity, or even go higher than we specify, if you dare.

1. Wash and sanitize all your fermentation equipment, including a knife and cutting board, and set aside to air-dry.

2. Make a salt brine by bringing 300 milliliters of the water to just under a boil in a small saucepan. Remove from the heat, add the salt, and stir well until all the salt has dissolved. Add the remaining 1,130 milliliters room-temperature water to the hot brine to cool it down; set aside.

3. Combine the carrots, lemon zest, lemon juice, and cayenne in the jar. Pour the kraut brine into the jar over the carrots. Pour the salt brine into the jar, leaving about 2 inches of headspace. Reserve the extra salt brine in a small jar in the refrigerator to use as needed. Seal the jar with the fermentation lid. Place the jar on a plate or in a bowl to catch any liquid displaced through the airlock during fermentation.

4. Ferment the carrot mixture in a cool place away from direct sunlight (2 weeks at 64°F is ideal—see the chart on page 287). Taste the carrot mixture after 1 week to determine if the sourness is to your liking. If it's not sour enough, reseal the jar and leave it to ferment for another week, then taste again.

5. When the carrot mixture is sour to your liking, strain it through a fine-mesh sieve set over a bowl; discard the carrots or reserve them for another use (see page 283). Transfer the liquid into bottles, seal, and store in the refrigerator for up to 6 months. Enjoy the carrot tonic still, or add flavoring and/or carbonation through a secondary fermentation in the bottle (see step 6 on page 329).

KAANJI

1,470 milliliters distilled or spring water

30 grams unrefined sea salt

390 grams sliced red or deep purple carrots (¼-inch-thick rounds)

1 tablespoon yellow or brown mustard seeds, coarsely ground using a mortar and pestle or spice grinder

100 milliliters natural brine from Basic Kraut (page 92) or 100 grams Basic Kraut

EQUIPMENT

Kitchen scale

½-gallon or 2-liter wide-mouth glass jar

Fermentation lid

3 pint jars

Kaanji is a traditional fermented beverage with roots in the Punjab region of India. This sour tonic is fermented in a saltier brine than our other sour tonics. Flavored with mustard seed, this delicious drink is traditionally used to aid digestion and replace salt lost by the body after a long day's work in the sweltering sun. We like both the red and dark purple varieties, but you can use any carrot, the color of which will be imparted to the finished beverage. To find these heirloom carrot varieties, you may have to pay a visit to your local farmers' market, where you are more likely to find carrot varieties in many different colors. Depending on what carrots you have access to, you can do as they do in India, substituting red beets for half the carrots if only light-colored carrots are available.

The fermented carrots left over after the liquid is strained are delicious, and can be eaten as a tangy snack or used as a salad topper.

1. Wash and sanitize all your fermentation equipment, including a knife and cutting board, and set aside to air-dry.

2. Make a salt brine by bringing 300 milliliters of the water to just under a boil in a small saucepan. Remove from the heat, add the salt, and stir well until all the salt has dissolved. Add the remaining 1,170 milliliters room-temperature water to the hot brine to cool it down; set aside.

3. Combine the carrots and mustard seeds in the jar. Pour the kraut brine into the jar over the carrots. Pour the salt brine into the jar, leaving about 2 inches of headspace. Reserve the extra salt brine in a small jar in the refrigerator to use as needed. Seal the jar with the fermentation lid. Place the jar on a plate or in a bowl to catch any liquid displaced through the airlock during fermentation.

4. Ferment the carrot mixture in a cool place away from direct sunlight (2 weeks at 64°F is ideal—see the chart on page 287). Taste the carrot mixture after 1 week to determine if the sourness is to your liking. If it's not sour enough, reseal the jar and leave it to ferment for another week, then taste again.

5. When the carrot mixture is sour to your liking, strain it through a fine-mesh sieve set over a bowl; discard the carrots or reserve them for another use (see page 283). Transfer the liquid into pint jars, seal, and store in the refrigerator for up to 10 months (longer than other sour tonics due to the higher salt content).

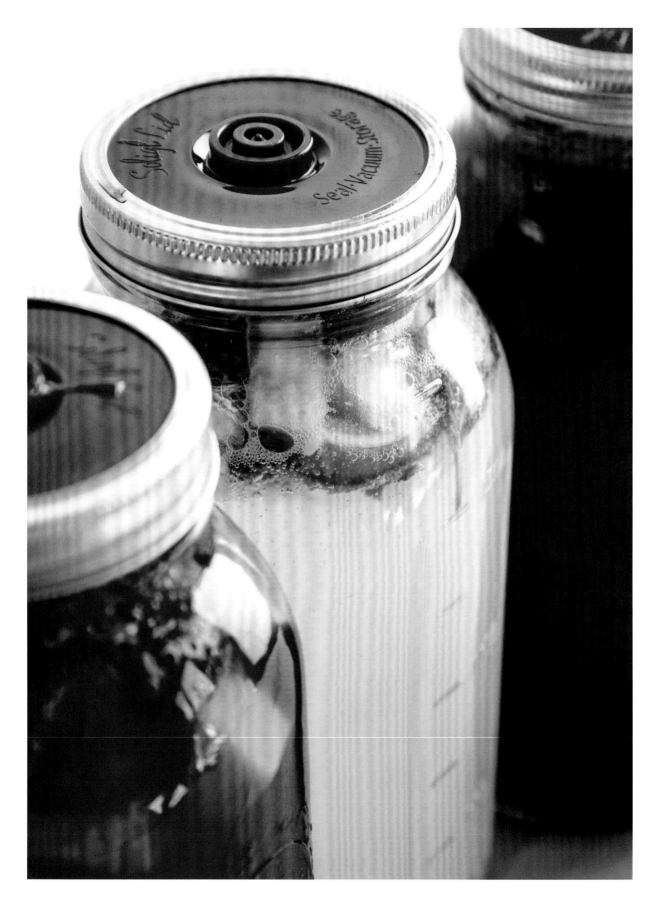

LIME-MINT CUCUMBER SOUR

MAKES ½ GALLON

1,390 milliliters distilled or spring water

10 grams unrefined sea salt

400 grams sliced cucumbers (½-inch-thick pieces)

1 tablespoon lime zest

100 milliliters lime juice (from 3 to 4 limes)

8 to 10 fresh mint sprigs, coarsely chopped

100 milliliters natural brine from Basic Kraut (page 92) or 100 grams Basic Kraut

EQUIPMENT

½-gallon or 2-liter wide-mouth glass jar

Fermentation lid

Kitchen scale

3 (16-ounce) bottles

In our neck of the woods, nothing says "summer" quite like a cold mojito at the beach. Incredibly refreshing with or without the rum, this is one sour tonic we definitely sweeten post-fermentation before serving over crushed ice.

Generally speaking, you don't need to peel the cucumbers, but if their skins are bitter, the flavor will ruin your tonic. Make sure to taste the skin before deciding.

If you're doing a secondary fermentation, you might consider adding just a bit of fresh mint to the bottles along with your sugar source, but we like this tonic just as much without bubbles.

1. Wash and sanitize all your fermentation equipment, including a knife and cutting board, and set aside to air-dry.

2. Make a salt brine by bringing 300 milliliters of the water to just under a boil in a small saucepan. Remove from the heat, add the salt, and stir well until all the salt has dissolved. Add the remaining 1,090 milliliters room-temperature water to the hot brine to cool it down; set aside.

3. Combine the cucumbers, lime zest, lime juice, and mint in the jar. Pour the kraut brine into the jar over the cucumbers. Pour the salt brine into the jar, leaving about 2 inches of headspace. Reserve the extra salt brine in a small jar in the refrigerator to use as needed. Seal the jar with the fermentation lid. Place the jar on a plate or in a bowl to catch any liquid displaced through the airlock during fermentation.

4. Ferment the cucumber mixture in a cool place away from direct sunlight (2 weeks at 64°F is ideal—see the chart on page 287). Taste the cucumber mixture after 1 week to determine if the sourness is to your liking. If it's not sour enough, reseal the jar and leave it to ferment for another week, then taste again.

5. When the cucumber mixture is sour to your liking, strain it through a fine-mesh sieve set over a bowl; discard the cucumbers (these leftover cucumbers do not make good fruit leather). Transfer the liquid into bottles, seal, and store in the refrigerator for up to 6 months. Enjoy the cucumber sour still, or add flavoring and/or carbonation through a secondary fermentation in the bottle (see step 6 on page 329).

Kombucha

Kombucha has become an iconic fermented beverage and has exploded on the US food scene over the past two decades. Although it has transcended the realm of "health fad" and become omnipresent on grocery store shelves nearly everywhere, it is by no means a new drink, and has been consumed by cultures around the world for thousands of years. Kombucha is believed to have originated in Manchuria, China, where it was prized during the Qin dynasty (221–206 BCE) for its energizing and detoxifying effects. It is conjectured that the culture traveled along the spice routes through Asia into what is now Russia and Eastern Europe, where it has a long tradition and is commonly called tea kvass. Throughout history, when humans have migrated to new lands, their cultural partners have migrated with them, spreading their microbial empire into new lands in symbiosis with their human hosts.

So what exactly *is* this magical healthy elixir? Kombucha is a mixture of tea, sugar, and water, fermented using a starter of previously acidified kombucha and a SCOBY (symbiotic culture of bacteria and yeast—see page 34). The kombucha SCOBY, also referred to as the kombucha mother, is a mat of cellulose woven on top of the tea mixture by the bacterium *Acetobacter xylinum*. This floating mat acts as a barrier and protects the fermenting liquid from the outside world while also drawing oxygen down into the liquid, to the benefit of the aerobic organisms. As the ferment progresses, a new SCOBY forms on top of the tea and will take the shape of your fermentation vessel. This means that each batch produces a new daughter SCOBY, which is used for the subsequent batch while the older mother SCOBY can be saved as a backup SCOBY or to be gifted to a fellow fermenter (we've given you some other ideas for using your SCOBYs on page 308). Someone is always in need of a SCOBY, even if they don't know it yet! So spread the SCOBYs to friends and family who are curious.

FERMENTER'S NOTES

Tea: Black tea is the tea most commonly used in kombucha, as it produces a lovely beverage with an almost apple cider flavor. The tea is oxidized, which contributes to its dark color and unique flavor. Green tea also makes a lovely kombucha; studies have shown that green tea has a stimulating effect on the kombucha SCOBY and, as a result, will ferment faster than black tea. We've kept it simple and just called for black tea in our kombucha recipe, but you can use black, green, white, oolong, and Pu-erh teas with great results. Just make sure they're pure teas, meaning they aren't flavored and contain no essential oils, which can be harmful to the SCOBY. We often use a combination of teas, such as equal parts white, green, and black. You can use loose tea leaves or an equal weight of tea bags (1 tea bag typically weighs between 1.5 and 2 grams).

Water: Good-quality spring or well water is ideal for making kombucha because it's full of minerals that are beneficial to the microbes and the fermentation. The tea and sugar do contain some nutrients and minerals, though, so filtered or distilled water can also be used with success. Just make sure that you never use unfiltered tap water from a municipal source, which contains chlorine and other chemicals that will be detrimental to the health of your culture.

Sugar: For kombucha you should use plain white sugar or cane sugar. Less refined sugars can be used, with varying effects, but in our view, cane sugar produces the best kombucha. Don't fret about the large quantity of sugar going into your brew, as almost all of it will be digested by the microbes and metabolized into acids and other by-products. The accepted range of sugar for kombucha is between 5 and 15% sugar by weight; our recipe uses to 10%. As the kombucha ferments, the yeasts digest the sugar and produce alcohol and CO_2, and then the bacteria convert the alcohol into acetic and gluconic acid. This means the more sugar you add in the beginning, the more acid will be present in the finished beverage, which will equate to a sourer flavor.

Culture: For this recipe, you'll need to obtain a SCOBY from a friend or buy one online (see Resources, page 348). Since every batch of kombucha produces a new SCOBY, it's typically easy to find someone with an extra SCOBY lying around (hopefully in a sweet tea "hotel"—more on that in a moment). You can also grow a kombucha SCOBY using store-bought kombucha. Some of my (Shane's) strongest and most active kombucha cultures have come from a bottle of GT's Living Foods kombucha. Their Classic Original flavor has higher alcohol content, but I have also had success using some of their flavored Original and Raw kombuchas. But all store-bought kombucha is not created equal—I've tried many other brands and have found that GT's seems to have the most active cultures in the bunch. To make your own SCOBY, divide the master formula recipe quantities in half (or even quarter them, to avoid wasting ingredients in case something goes wrong and the batch doesn't form a mother), prepare the batch, and at the point where you normally place the kombucha mother in the jar, pour in a bottle of store-bought kombucha instead. Let it ferment until the kombucha is quite acidic and a thick mother has formed on top, then use the mother and the acidified liquid as the starter culture for making a full batch. Store any leftover acidified kombucha in the refrigerator and use it for one of its many uses (see page 308). If a mother doesn't form within two weeks, it probably isn't going to happen, and you should toss the failed batch and try another brand of bottled kombucha.

You can store many kombucha mothers in a "SCOBY hotel," a dedicated jar or vessel for your backup SCOBY stock. To start a hotel, simply follow the recipe for Kombucha on page 306, submerge your backup SCOBYs in the liquid, and cover with a porous cloth. A new SCOBY will form on top of the hotel creating a nice barrier that will protect the backups submerged below. Keep the hotel at room temperature and simply refresh it with a little sweet tea every time you make a new batch of kombucha, which will give the SCOBYs sugar to eat so they stay alive and active. SCOBY hotels can withstand quite a bit of neglect, lasting many months in cooler weather without feeding, but if neglected for too long, the liquid will turn so acidic that the culture will die and your backup SCOBYs will essentially be pickled.

The master formula recipe that follows yields 3½ liters but is designed to be made in a 1-gallon or 4-liter vessel, which allows space for the new SCOBY to grow on top. You don't want to fill the vessel to the top because you need to allow space for the kombucha mother to grow, and you want the new mother to form at the vessel's widest point. If you fill the vessel all the way to the top, where most jars are narrower, the new mother will form to that diameter. Then as you drink or pull samples of the kombucha (lowering the level of the liquid), the mother will no longer cover the entire surface of the liquid, which can result in contamination or the SCOBY sinking from its protective position on top. Having a fermentation vessel with a spigot on it really helps to access the liquid for tasting without disturbing the floating mother on the surface.

Fermenting: Maintaining a temperature of 70°F in your house can be difficult, especially in the winter. In low temperatures, kombucha can take a very long time to ferment, sometimes as long as three months. The opposite is true of warm temperatures, in which the kombucha will ferment much faster. If fermenting under cooler conditions, it is advantageous to use a seedling starting mat to raise the ambient temperature around the fermentation vessel by about 10°F. See page 81 for more information on DIY fermentoriums and how to maintain temperature.

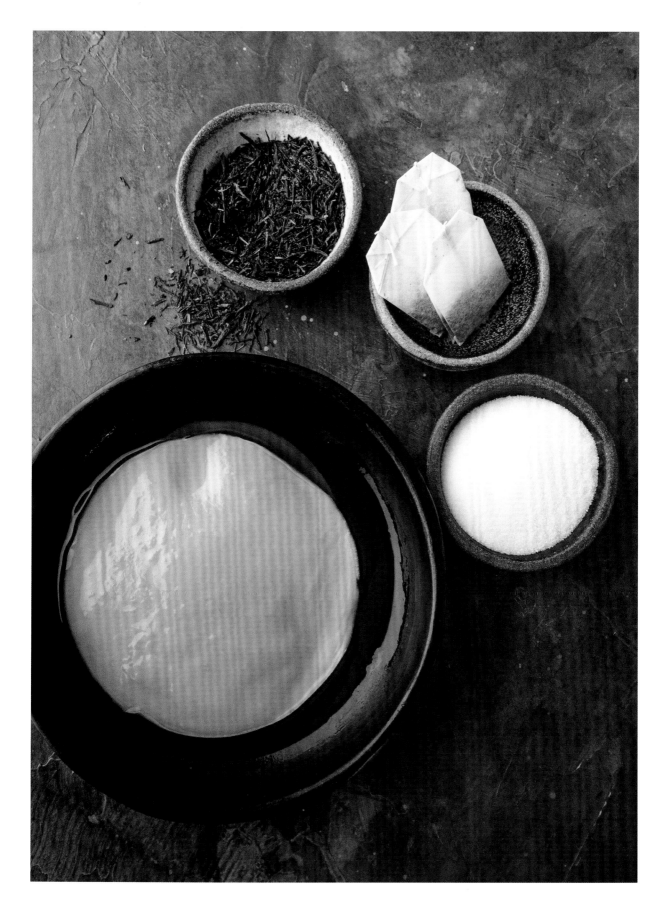

SOUR KOMBUCHA OR KOMBUCHA VINEGAR

Along with the excess SCOBYs, your home kombucha production will also yield overly sour kombucha from time to time. It is inevitable that occasionally a batch of kombucha will be left to ferment for too long, yielding a very sour liquid that more resembles vinegar than it does a tasty kombucha. In fact, overfermented kombucha liquid can become so tart that it is no longer palatable as a beverage, but don't throw this sour liquid out! Sour kombucha, also called kombucha vinegar (for obvious reasons), can essentially be used as a vinegar substitute in your home cooking. We love kombucha vinegar in salad dressings (replace half the vinegar in any salad dressing with kombucha vinegar), for finishing soups, or in Kombucha Mayo. Another great culinary use for kombucha vinegar is to make kombucha shrub syrups, a fruit-infused sour syrup used as the base for refreshing alcoholic or nonalcoholic beverages.

Finally, kombucha vinegar has other uses outside of the kitchen—believe it or not it makes an excellent conditioning hair rinse! Simply apply kombucha vinegar to wet hair in the shower, work it in, and rinse. You can also use it in foot soaks, creams, and face masks. The versatility of the kombucha vinegar and its myriad uses make this sour liquid an excellent ingredient for those who are into home remedies and home apothecary. If you decide to use your kombicha culture for cosmetic purposes, just be sure to keep the liquid and SCOBYs in a dedicated vessel labeled as "cosmetic," to avoid cross-contaminating with the cultures you are using for culinary purposes.

MAKES ABOUT 1¼ CUPS

2 egg yolks, at room temperature

1 tablespoon kombucha vinegar

1 teaspoon champagne or
white wine vinegar

½ teaspoon Dijon mustard

235 milliliters grapeseed oil

½ teaspoon salt

MAKES ABOUT 1½ PINTS
SYRUP, FOR 15 TO
20 COCKTAILS

250 grams stemmed fresh
whole strawberries or any
other fruit, muddled

700 milliliters kombucha vinegar

Sugar equivalent to half of liquid
yield, see recipe

Vodka (optional)

Soda water and ice for serving

Kombucha Mayo

We've been making mayonnaise with kraut liquid for years but for this book we decided to try a version with kombucha. We're glad we did because we found that we preferred the rounded, smooth flavors of this slightly sweeter version.

Combine all ingredients in a 1-pint or ½-liter jar and blend with an immersion blender for 20 seconds. Seal the jar and store in the refrigerator. The mayonnaise will firm up in the refrigerator and will keep for about a week.

Strawberry Kombucha Shrub

You can make kombucha shrubs with any type of fruit. Berries are an excellent option because they are so juicy, easy to muddle, and therefore easily infused into the kombucha vinegar. If using other fruits besides berries, you might need to chop them up instead of muddling to get a good infusion. Kombucha shrub cocktails or mocktails are pleasantly refreshing on a warm day, with a nice balance between sweet and sour.

Combine the muddled berries and kombucha vinegar in a 1-quart or 1-liter jar, cover with a loose-fitting lid or cheesecloth secured in place, and allow the fruit to infuse into the liquid for 2 to 3 days at room temperature. Strain the liquid into a bowl through a fine-mesh sieve and discard the solids. Measure the amount of liquid you have yielded in grams, and combine the liquid with a quantity of sugar equal to half the quantity of liquid yielded, in a medium pot. Bring the mixture to a boil, uncovered, over medium-high heat, stirring frequently until the sugar is dissolved. Lower the heat and simmer for about an hour, until syrupy. Remove from the heat, allow the shrub syrup to cool slightly, and pour into smaller jars or bottles. Store the shrub in the refrigerator, where it will last for up to a year.

For a shrub cocktail, combine one part vodka (or your preferred liquor) to one part shrub syrup over ice, and top with soda water. For a shrub mocktail, simply fill a glass almost to the top with soda water and ice and add the shrub syrup to taste.

KOMBUCHA

MAKES ABOUT 3½ QUARTS

2,800 milliliters spring or distilled water

15 grams loose-leaf black tea or black tea bags

350 grams sugar

350 milliliters acidified kombucha (from a previous batch, or use store-bought— see Fermenter's Notes, page 301)

1 SCOBY mother

EQUIPMENT

Kitchen scale

Stainless-steel or plastic fine-mesh sieve

1-gallon/4-liter jar or crock (one with a spigot is optimal)

6 (16-ounce) bottles

I'll never forget the first time I encountered a kombucha culture floating in a jar on a friend's kitchen counter. It was unlike anything I'd ever seen— more like an alien blob than anything meant to be ingested by humans. With post-Pasteurian apprehension but propelled by my curiosity, I "drank the Kool-Aid," so to speak, and was immediately hooked by the deliciously refreshing, effervescent tang. One of the things I love most about making my own kombucha is the communal aspect of propagating and sharing the culture with others. My first SCOBY, which I perpetuated for years, was given to me by a friend. Many years later, when that same friend lost her SCOBY to neglect, I gave her a SCOBY from the same cultural lineage as the one she had gifted to me. —Shane

1. Wash and sanitize all your fermentation equipment and set aside to air-dry.

2. Weigh out the total quantity of water. I like to use a 1-gallon plastic water jug for this task, to which you can draw a watermark line in permanent marker in order to streamline the process for future batches.

3. Bring 800 milliliters of the water to a boil in a medium pot. Remove the pot from the heat and add the tea leaves or bags. Cover with a tight-fitting lid and set aside to steep for 15 minutes. Strain the tea through the fine-mesh sieve into a large pot or bowl, pressing down on the tea leaves or bags with a wooden spoon to extract as much liquid as possible; discard the tea leaves or bags.

4. Add the sugar to the hot tea and stir until the sugar has completely dissolved. Add the remaining 2,000 milliliters room-temperature water to the tea to cool it down and stir to combine. (Cooling the tea makes it safe for the live cultures in the SCOBY and acidified kombucha, as hot liquid can harm them. Slightly warmer than room temperature is acceptable, but if the mixture is too hot when you add the SCOBY and acidified kombucha, it could result in a failed batch. Play it safe so you don't harm your kombucha culture!)

5. Transfer the room-temperature sweet tea to the jar. Add the acidified kombucha and stir to combine.

6. Gently place the kombucha mother in the jar on top of the liquid. (Don't worry if it sinks to the bottom initially; it should at least partially float back up to the top as the mixture ferments, and a new SCOBY will form on the surface of the liquid within the first week. If the mother does not float to the top and a new SCOBY fails to form, your culture is not viable and you'll need to start over.)

7. Cover the jar with a piece of fine-mesh cheesecloth, a clean piece of cotton fabric, or a paper towel and secure it with a rubber band or clean kitchen twine.

8. Ferment the kombucha in a warm place completely away from direct sunlight (2 weeks at 75°F is ideal—see the chart at right). Take care to not jostle or move the vessel too much during fermentation, or else the new SCOBY that forms on top could be disturbed and sink to the bottom, which can result in surface contamination.

9. Taste the fermenting kombucha often, starting once you can clearly see new SCOBY forming and thickening on top, at around day 7, to gauge the acidity, effervescence, and level of sweetness in the liquid. (This is where a vessel with a spigot comes in handy, because it enables you to taste the kombucha without disturbing the mother.) The key to making good kombucha is to bottle it at the right point;

the point in time when the beverage is balanced between sweet, sour, and a slight effervescence. Often, this "sweet spot" only lasts a couple days; if it's missed, you will have a sour beverage, and it will be more difficult, though not impossible, to carbonate. Everyone has a different preference as to sweetness and acidity, so go by your preference there, but keep a close taste bud on the level of effervescence as well. Bottling your kombucha right at the point when the effervescence has peaked, almost fizzled out, but yet is still detectable, will offer a better chance at carbonating your kombucha through a secondary fermentation in the bottle.

10. When the kombucha is ready, transfer it into bottles, seal, and store in the refrigerator for up to 6 months. Enjoy the kombucha as is, or add flavoring and/or carbonation through a secondary fermentation in the bottle (see step 6 on page 329).

Fermentation Temperature & Time
Above 80°F Ferment 1 week or less
76° to 80°F Ferment 1 to 2 weeks
Ideal: 75°F Ferment 2 weeks
70° to 74°F Ferment 2 to 3 weeks
Below 70°F Ferment 3 weeks or more

THE EVER-USEFUL SCOBY

When you start making kombucha, the SCOBYs can multiply quite rapidly and, before you know it, you'll have too many to deal with. But oh, the things you can do with a SCOBY! There are too many uses to list, but here is a collection of some of our favorite things to do with your excess SCOBYs.

Nata: I have to admit that sour candy is one of my guilty pleasures. I know those little chewy pieces of corn syrup laced with citric acid and food coloring are just about the worst thing I could be eating, but hey, we all have our things. If you share my affinity for sour, sugary, chewy goodness, then nata might just be for you. It's a great alternative to sour candy with a pleasingly tart and almost applelike fruitiness you would not expect to find from a kombucha mother. To make nata, chop a roughly 1-inch-thick SCOBY into bite-size pieces. Combine the chopped SCOBY and a roughly equal quantity of sugar in a medium saucepan and bring the mixture to a boil over medium-high heat, stirring constantly until the sugar melts. Cook the SCOBY chunks in the syrup that forms for about 15 minutes, stirring often. Remove from the heat and allow the mixture to cool. Use a slotted spoon to remove the pieces of SCOBY from the syrup and place them on dehydrator sheets or a baking sheet. Dehydrate the pieces in a dehydrator at 150°F for 2 to 3 hours or in the oven on the lowest heat setting; keep an eye on the nata and remove it from the oven while it's still chewy, before it fully hardens. The texture of the finished nata should be close to gummy candy. Store the nata in an airtight container at room temperature, where it will keep quite well for a very long time if you dehydrated the candy sufficiently. I had some nata that I had forgotten about in the back of a cupboard and it was still good after over a year of being stored at room temperature.

Some prefer to boil the nata in water for 15 minutes prior to cooking it with the sugar to remove some of its acidity. Another variation is to sprinkle the nata with additional sugar just prior to dehydrating. If you are averse to using sugar, you can boil the nata in fruit juice or coconut water instead of sugar, which will also add flavor to the finished nata.

Face Mask: Believe it or not SCOBYs make a lovely face mask! As Hannah Crum states on her website, Kombucha Kamp, "It will pull circulation to the face, which regenerates skin cells. The pH will create a mild acid peel which sloughs away dead skin and the cellulose structure creates nano-structures that help to fill in fine lines and wrinkles." You can apply one of your thinner SCOBYs directly to your face as a mask, or you can make a kombucha cream: Combine roughly equal parts acidified kombucha liquid and coarsely chopped pieces of SCOBY in a blender. Blend until somewhat smooth (some small SCOBY chunks will still be visible), adding more liquid kombucha if needed to reach a creamy texture. This cream can be spread on the face for a mask, used as a topical

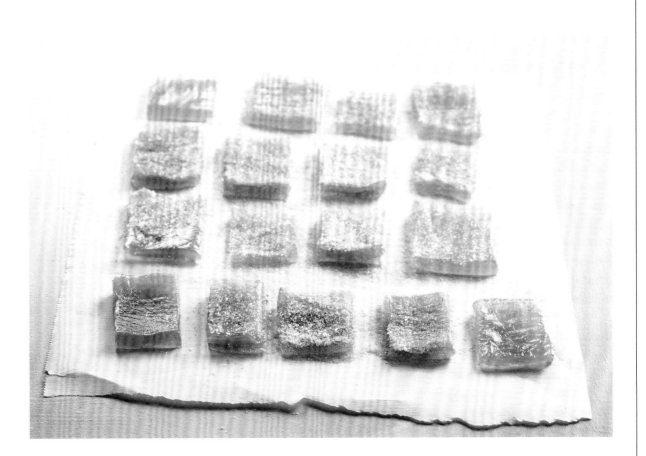

remedy for skin maladies, or applied to wounds as a poultice. You can also mix liquid kombucha with clay and honey to make another face mask. I keep a jar of SCOBY chunks in acidified kombucha liquid in my refrigerator to be used for just cosmetic purposes.

Living Band-Aid: This is one of our favorite uses for the kombucha mother. Cosmetic companies are actually starting to market and sell "living Band-Aids," essentially utilizing the same organism that makes the kombucha SCOBY. Simply slice a small, thin piece of kombucha mother to fit the wound you want to cover, place the "living Band-Aid" over the wound, stretch it slightly, and allow it to dry. It will actually blend in well with your skin, making the wound less noticeable. The living bandage will create a SCOBY scab that allows oxygen to reach the wound, which will speed up the healing process. The healthy acids from the kombucha also help to heal the wound.

—Shane

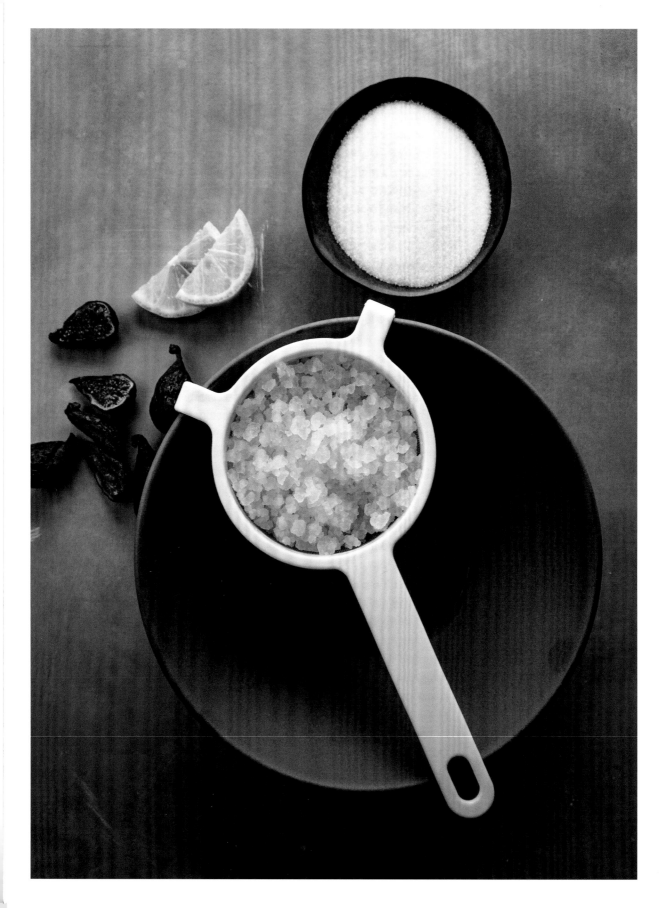

48 hours! Once the culture has doubled to 120 grams, you can either divide the grains between two 1-quart or 1-liter jars, or scale your batches up to ½ gallon or 2 liters by simply doubling the master formula recipe. If your kefir grains are not adequately growing in mass with each new batch, use the coconut-mango variation on page 316; the mineral-rich coconut water causes explosive growth in the kefir grains and is a great recipe for doubling up your grains if you're trying to scale up your kefir batch size. The grains need to fed consistently, about every two to three days, to remain viable. If you leave them unattended for an extended duration, the liquid will become too acidic and the grains will lose viability and disintegrate into nothing. If you're going on vacation, or simply want to put the culture "on hold," you can dehydrate the grains in the sun or in a dehydrator set to low (below 100°F), and then store them in a plastic bag in the refrigerator for up to a year. Drying in the sun is our preferred method. Simply spread the grains out on a baking sheet or cutting board, set in a sunny place, and check every 2 hours until the grains are dry. Finally, you can also seal the grains in a plastic bag and put them in the freezer, where they will keep for 6 months or more.

Fermenting: In warm weather, water kefir can ferment very fast. Increasing the sugar in the initial mixture will give the grains more food, allowing the culture to survive longer in warm temperatures as well as giving you longer between feedings. This increased sugar will also result in a more acidic finished beverage, so taste often if fermenting in warm weather. Do not increase the sugar much past 15%. Alternatively, if your kefir grains are slow to ferment, you can decrease the sugar, or you can add 10% liquid from a previous batch to speed up fermentation.

Flavoring: We've found that the easiest way to flavor water kefir is to make an unflavored batch, then use dried or fresh fruit, fruit juice, or flavored syrup (see pages 345 to 347) to prime the bottles before a secondary fermentation. This method adds flavor and will also help to carbonate the kefir, giving the microbes more sugar to digest. If using dried fruit during the primary fermentation, it can be annoyingly difficult to separate the grains from the fruit, post-fermentation. However, you can use a spice bag to keep the fruit and grains separate, or simply tie the dried fruit in a piece of cheesecloth.

SWISS-STYLE WATER KEFIR

MAKES 1 QUART

675 milliliters spring or distilled water

75 grams sugar

20 grams dried figs (1 or 2)

10 grams dried raisins

1 thin slice of lemon

60 grams active water kefir grains

FLAVORING OPTIONS
(PER 16-OUNCE BOTTLE)

20 grams dried fruit

50 to 100 milliliters pure fruit juice

1 tablespoon fruit syrup or herb-infused syrup (see pages 345 to 347)

1 teaspoon corn sugar (see Notes) or other sugar

EQUIPMENT

Kitchen scale

1-quart or 1-liter glass jar

Stainless-steel or plastic fine-mesh sieve

2 (16-ounce) flip-top glass bottles or bottles of your choice, for storage

There are numerous variations of water kefir from around the world, owing to the spread of the kefir grain culture around the globe at various points in history. This variation has been adapted from a Swiss recipe for water kefir and has become one of our go-to recipes for this beverage. The figs and raisins both add minerals to the mixture, along with flavor and another sugar source for the microbes. The lemon slice adds just a hint of acidity and lemon flavor to the finished beverage. You can make your own water kefir variations utilizing many different sugars, dried fruits, and fruit juices as the base for the fermentation. We offer you two well-tested variations below, but this ferment is really fun to experiment with, and changing the sugar source or the type of dried fruit can really change the profile of the finished beverage.

1. Wash and sanitize all your fermentation equipment and set aside to air-dry.

2. Bring 100 milliliters of the water to just under a boil in a small saucepan. Remove from the heat, add the sugar, and stir until all the sugar has dissolved.

3. Add the figs, raisins, and lemon slice to the hot sugar water and let stand for 5 minutes (this infuses the sugar water with flavor and also helps to minimize any microbes the fruit may be harboring). Pour the mixture into the jar and add the remaining 575 milliliters of room-temperature water to cool it down. Stir to combine. Add the water kefir grains to the jar. The grains will sink to the bottom of the vessel, where they will work their magic.

4. Cover the jar with either a piece of cheesecloth or a clean paper towel and secure it with a metal screw band or a rubber band. Ferment the water kefir in a warm place such as in a cupboard in a warm part of your house or on top of the refrigerator (3 days at 68°F is ideal—see the chart opposite). Taste the water kefir after 2 days. You should see bubbles floating up to the top from the culture below.

5. When the water kefir is slightly sour but still slightly sweet and has a touch of effervescence, strain it through the fine-mesh sieve set over a bowl or pitcher. (Be sure the sieve is stainless steel or plastic, as some metals will react to the acidity in the kefir, and can impart metallic flavors.) Set the kefir aside. Discard the figs and lemon slice

and set the grains aside in the sieve (keep an eye on them—you don't want them to dry out).

6. Prime the bottles, meaning add a sugar source to the bottle, with one of the flavoring options. Pour the kefir into the bottles and seal. Let the bottles sit out at room temperature to allow for a secondary fermentation, 1 to 3 days, depending on temperature (see Notes). To gauge the level of carbonation you can gently lift the flip-top on one of the bottles; if CO_2 has been produced and the bottles have successfully been carbonated, a little gas will escape when you flip the top. Alternatively, you can bottle one of your kefir bottles in plastic, which allows you to gauge the carbonation by squeezing the bottle and feeling the resistance (as the beverage becomes carbonated, the bottle will become more resistant and quite firm when squeezed). Once carbonated, move the bottles to the refrigerator and enjoy

within 3 weeks. Even in refrigeration, the kefir will continue to ferment and build pressure in the bottle, depending on how much residual sugar is in the bottle. Take extra care to not forget about bottles of water kefir in your fridge, as it could lead to exploding bottles.

7. After you've bottled your first batch of water kefir, you can begin a second batch, or follow the instructions on page 313 to put your kefir grains on hold. To start another batch, make the sugar water as directed and add the grains from the sieve. (If the kefir grains have formed an excessive white film, rinse them with fresh water, but otherwise they do not need to be rinsed.) We typically get into a rhythm where we always have a batch fermenting, a batch carbonating on the counter, and a finished batch in the fridge.

CONTINUED >

Fermentation Temperature & Time

Above 72°F
Ferment 2 days or less

69° to 72°F
Ferment 2 to 3 days

Ideal: 68°F
Ferment 3 days

64° to 67°F
Ferment 3 to 4 days

Below 64°F
Ferment 4 days or more

Notes: Corn sugar is commonly used by brewers because it is fine grained and dissolves easily in liquid. It's widely available at brewing supply stores.

Caution! Water kefir can be a very active culture. Overcarbonation is a real thing, and if your water kefir gets too carbonated, it can result in exploding bottles, at worst, or the beverage spouting up like a geyser when the bottle is opened, resulting in most of the beverage being lost (probably all over you and your kitchen). Read the section on flavoring and carbonating beverages (see page 342) before beginning this secondary fermentation.

Variations

Date-Orange Water Kefir

675 milliliters purified or spring water

75 grams coconut sugar

20 grams coarsely chopped pitted dried dates

1 orange slice

60 grams active water kefir grains

Follow the instructions in the master formula, substituting the coconut sugar for the sugar, the dates for the figs and raisins, and the orange slice for the lemon.

Coconut-Mango Water Kefir

175 milliliters purified or spring water

50 grams sugar

20 grams dried mango

500 milliliters pure 100% coconut water

60 grams active water kefir grains

Follow the instructions in the master formula but heat the total amount of water (175 milliliters), add the sugar and mango, stir to dissolve the sugar, and use the coconut water to cool the mixture down prior to adding the water kefir culture.

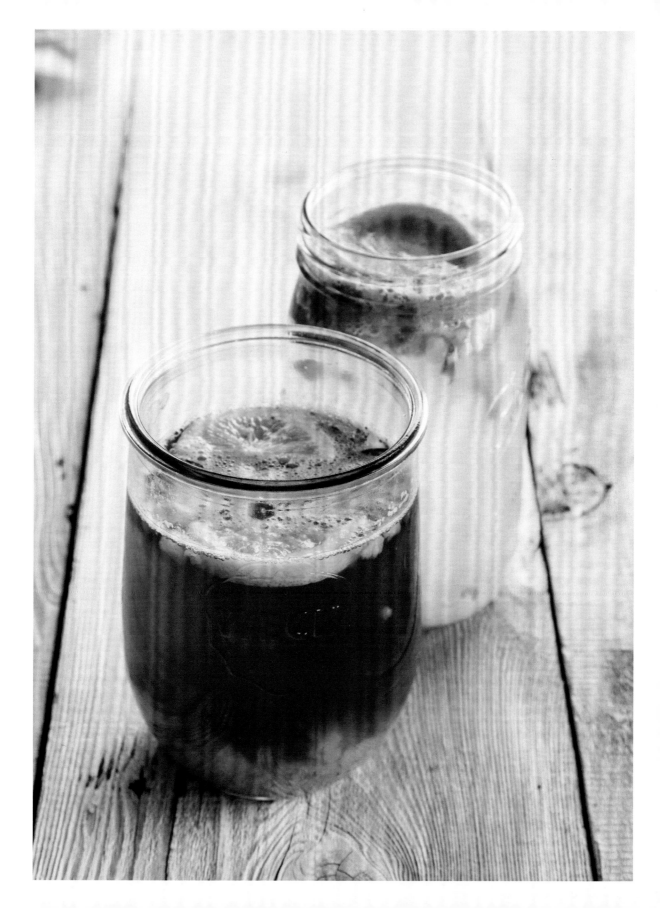

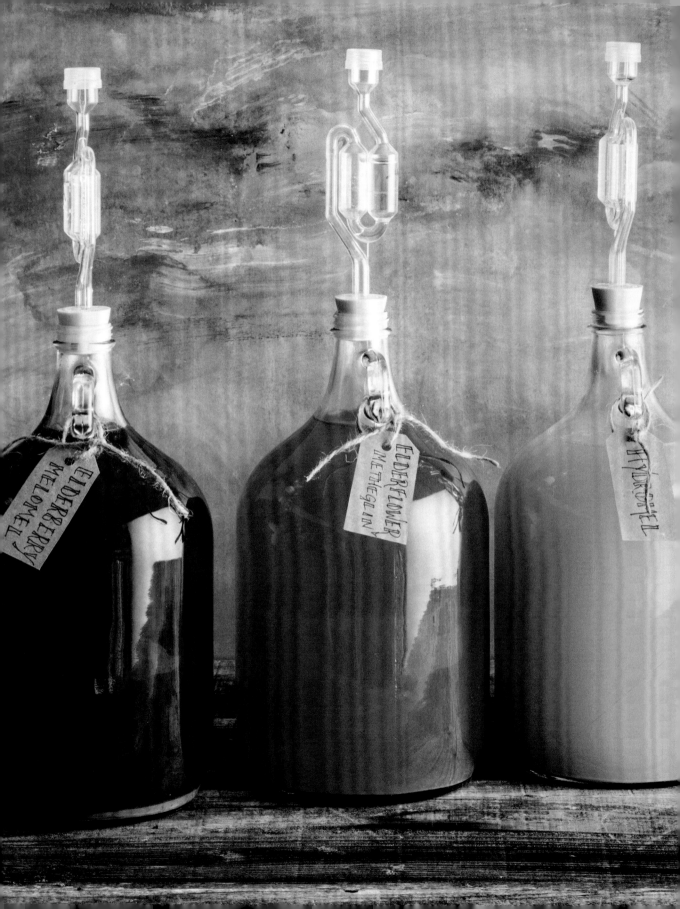

Meads

The story of fermented honey, commonly called mead around the world, is deeply and intricately interwoven into the fabric of our ancestral history. Also called honey wine, nectar of the gods, or ambrosia, mead has been produced by nearly every culture that has had access to honey, and it was central to the spirituality and mythology of our ancient ancestors. In many ancient cultures, mead was considered sacred, a gift from the gods, with the ability to change the consciousness of those who consumed it. Along with the sacred aspect of mead, it was considered a life-enhancing health elixir, and was also a major source of sustenance. The earliest evidence of mead production dates all the way back to 7000 BCE, in China, where pottery vessels containing residue from a fermented beverage made with rice, honey, and fruit have been found. Since mead is most likely the first alcohol fermented by humans, it seemed only proper to include it in this book.

I (Shane) have been a steward of bees for about seven years at the time of this writing. My love of bees and beekeeping led me on the journey to mead making, which I have enjoyed immensely for many years. But it wasn't until I read *Sacred and Herbal Healing Beers* by Stephen Harrod Buhner that I really fell in love with mead making. His book is fascinating, and I highly recommend it to anyone interested in the subject. To quote him here, "Mead is the fermentation of honey, producing a liquor that allows human beings, for a time, to experience sacred states of mind. And more, all three things—bees, honey, and mead—confer on humankind some of the immortality of the gods, giving them long life, health, and a deepening of consciousness and awareness." I know that this has been true for me, as caring for and loving the bees, respecting their gifts, and making mead have all raised my level of consciousness and brought me closer to the natural world, and my own true nature.

Bees are such amazing little creatures, and we have reached a point where they need our love, respect, and stewardship more than ever. Honey is an expensive ingredient, both in the price it demands and the expense of labor for the bees to produce it. Cherish and respect the bees and the amazing honey they produce. Next time you are blessed with the gift of honey (because it is most definitely a precious gift), remember that it takes the bees visiting about 2 million flowers or 55,000 miles of flight to produce 1 pound of honey! (To put that in perspective, to make our basic hydromel, which calls for 2 pounds of honey, a colony of bees would have to make the equivalent of about four trips around the earth at the equator.) If that's not extraordinary, and reason enough to respect and love the bees, I don't know what is.

Mead can be flavored with dried fruit, fruit juices, spices, and herbs. There are many misconceptions about mead, mainly that it is an overly sweet dessert wine. Indeed, most commercially available meads are, in fact, overly sweet dessert wines (properly called sack meads or sack), but the mead-making possibilities amount to much more than that. Meads can range from sweet to semisweet, but they can also be fermented to the point that they are so dry and effervescent, they resemble a Champagne. Depending on the ratio of honey to water used and the prevalent microbial cultures, the alcohol content can range drastically from a lightly alcoholic 3 to 4 percent to a highly inebriating 20 percent. The addition of many different medicinal and culinary herbs can increase the mead's inebriating qualities, enhance the fermentation, and act as preservatives. There are hundreds of different types of meads, and it is not possible to discuss them all in this book.

The greatest defining influences on mead making are the variety of honey used, the ratio of water to honey, the handling and preparation of the raw ingredients, and the type of yeast and/or bacteria present in the must. Mead is meant to be aged for at least 6 months before it's enjoyed, though a year is even better.

> *"Mead is the ancient liquor of gods and men, the giver of knowledge and poetry, the healer of wounds, and the bestower of immortality."*
>
> —ROBERT GAYRE, 1948

FERMENTER'S NOTES

Honey: The more honey you use, the higher the alcohol content of the finished product will be. By using more or less honey, and depending on the yeast strain you use, you can make any of the meads in this chapter still or sparkling, sweet or dry. The honey you choose will have a huge impact on the final flavor of the beverage, especially with hydromels, which consist of only honey, water, and yeast and really put the variety of honey on display. In California, I prefer spring wildflower honeys for hydromels; these varieties are typically light and floral, whereas some of the more pungent and

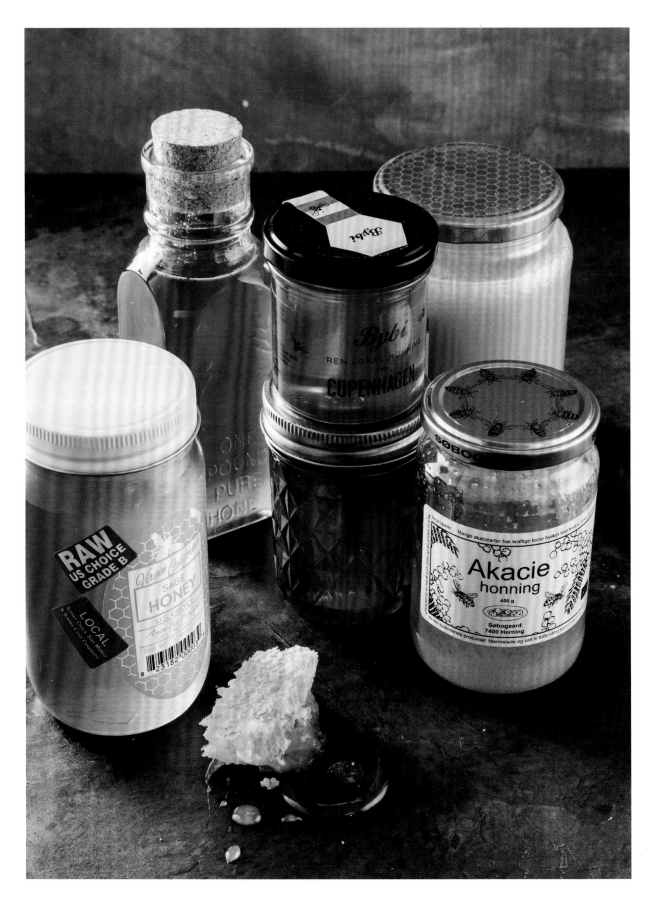

darker late-summer/fall honeys are too overpowering and are more appropriate for metheglins (herbal-infused meads). In the West, our fall honeys can be quite pungent, with madrone and other late-blooming trees adding bitter notes. I find these notes are balanced and partially covered up by the addition of herbs. The advantage of using a darker, late-season honey is that they typically have a higher mineral content, which can have a beneficial effect on fermentation and result in a shorter fermentation time. Some other light, floral honey varietals that are great for hydromels are acacia, clover, orange blossom, heather, lavender, sage, and star thistle, to name a few.

Even though most mead makers will tell you to heat the honey, I advise a no-heat method, primarily because heating honey can degrade the volatile compounds that deliver flavor and aroma, resulting in a less flavorful mead. Also, the main reason mead makers heat their honey is to kill any wild microbes that may be present, but if you use a healthy yeast starter, it will outcompete the wild strains in the honey.

If your honey is crystallized, heat the jar in a pot of warm water to melt it sufficiently to facilitate dissolving it into the water.

Sugar: You can use any sugar as a priming sugar, but corn sugar is commonly used by brewers because it is fine grained and dissolves easily in liquid. It's widely available at brewing supply stores. I use corn sugar for priming beers, but I typically use honey to prime my meads.

Specific gravity: Specific gravity is a measurement of the amount of dissolved solids in a medium (in this case, honey/sugars dissolved in water) and is used to calculate ABV (alcohol by volume); it's also used to help determine when to bottle your mead. A small handheld device called a hydrometer (see page 53) is used to measure gravity. Here is a rough guide to the desired finished gravity (FG) of each style of mead.

Dry meads: 0.990 to 1.006
Medium meads: 1.006 to 1.015
Sweet meads: 1.012 to 1.020
Dessert meads: 1.020 and higher

To figure out the ABV of your finished mead, find an online calculator and enter the original gravity (OG) and FG of the mead.

Yeast: Traditionally, meads were fermented using wild yeast and bacteria, both of which are present in raw honey, as well as on the skins of fruit. Relying on the naturally occurring bacteria and yeast in raw honey can produce very fine, nuanced meads, but it can also be inconsistent and produce some funky off-flavors that you might find to be unappealing. Yeast is relatively cheap (around $1 per packet, which typically cultures up to

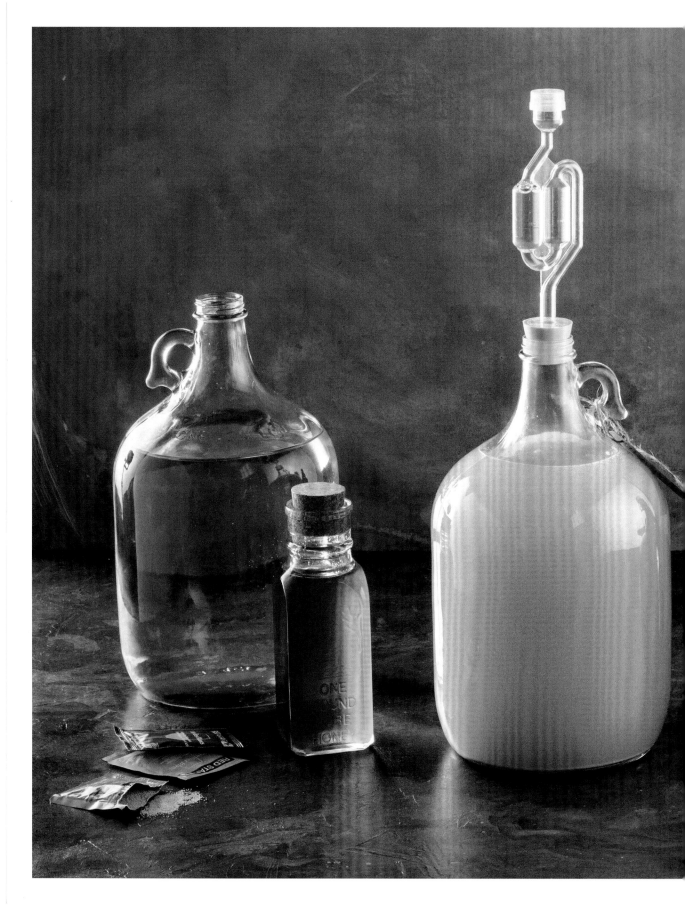

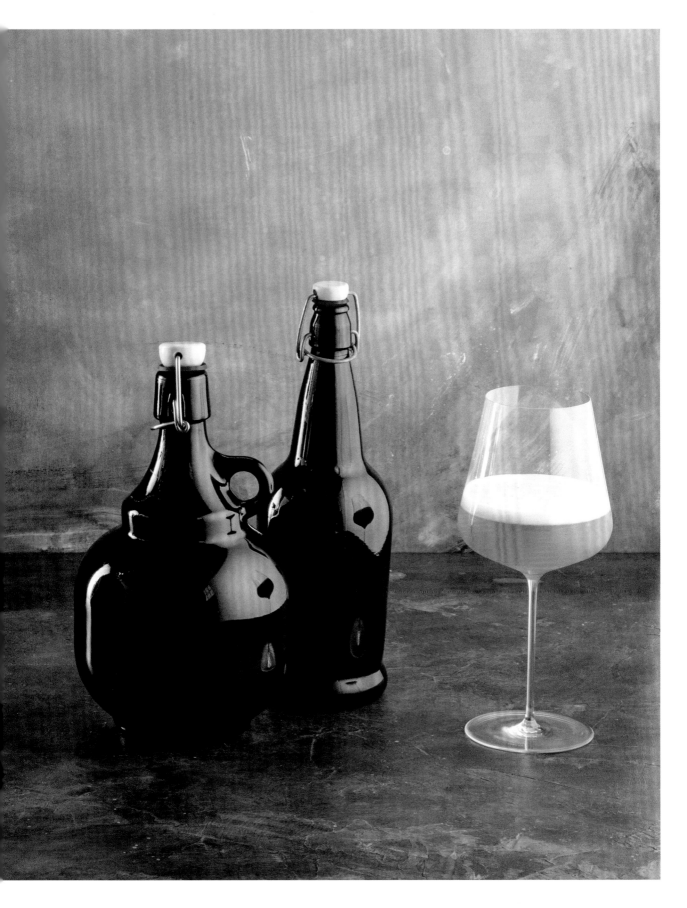

DRY SPARKLING MEAD (BASIC HYDROMEL)

MAKES 1 GALLON

50 milliliters warm filtered water (85° to 95°F)

1 packet (5 grams) Lalvin EC-1118 Champagne yeast (see Note) or a comparable Champagne yeast

1,000 grams floral spring honey or other variety (see page 321)

3,200 milliliters filtered water

2 grams BSG CraftBrewing Superfood or a comparable yeast nutrient

Honey or sugar (see pages 321, 323), for priming the bottles

EQUIPMENT

Hydrometer

1-gallon carboy with rubber bung (size 6.5) and airlock

Funnel or siphon

4 (1-quart or 1-liter) flip-top glass bottles or bottles of your choice, for aging

There's nothing quite as beautiful as a basic hydromel (water and honey) made from a floral honey varietal. While the bees' process of evaporation renders the water content of honey so low (around 17 percent) that organisms such as yeast cannot ferment it, raw honey will ferment spontaneously once water is added. This tendency for raw honey to naturally and spontaneously ferment was no doubt how humans developed this fermented honey wine far before other types of fermentations. The common scenario put forth is something like this: Many thousands of years ago, a tree containing a colony of bees splintered in a storm, the combs were broken and the honey collected in a natural basin, and was then diluted with rainwater. The honey water, full of yeasts, naturally started to ferment. Then a human came along and found this beautiful and intoxicating liquid—and the rest is history. When sipping hydromels, I like to imagine this scenario and think of the first human who encountered this golden fermented liquid in the wild and had the courage to drink it. What thoughts must have raced through their minds upon tasting such a hydromel, beautifully crafted by nature.

I prefer to make my hydromels dry and sparkling like this one, but you can also make them sweet to medium, and still to slightly effervescent. If you want a sweeter mead, simply ferment for less time, bottling before the mead ferments to dryness, or increase the honey in the initial recipe, bottle the mead without priming the bottles, and immediately move the bottles to cellar temperature (50° to 60°F) or into the refrigerator. You can also try using Wyeast sweet mead yeast (4184) instead of the Lalvin EC-1118. —Shane

1. Wash and sanitize all your fermentation equipment and set aside to air-dry.

2. To hydrate the yeast, put the 50 milliliters warm water in a measuring cup and pour in the powdered yeast. Let the yeast and warm water stand for 10 to 15 minutes, then stir to combine. (If using a different style of yeast, such as liquid yeast, follow the instructions on the package.)

3. Combine the honey and the 3,200 milliliters water in a large stockpot. Add the hydrated yeast and stir to combine. Add the yeast nutrient to the must and stir to combine. Using a wooden spoon, stir vigorously for 5 minutes (this oxygenates the must, which will facilitate the growth of the yeast). Alternatively, transfer some of the must to a blender and blend

for a few minutes to incorporate oxygen, then return the blended must to the pot.

4. Measure the specific gravity of the unfermented must (this is the original gravity, or OG). Fill the hydrometer test tube about three-quarters full with must, place the hydrometer in the tube of must, and spin it with your fingers. It will bob and eventually settle. Make a note of this number. Transfer the must to the carboy using either the funnel or siphon, leaving the neck of the carboy empty, or leaving 3 to 4 inches of headspace.

5. Ferment the mead in a warm place away from direct sunlight (4 weeks at 70°F is ideal—see the chart at right). Check the bung during the first couple of days, as the pressure building inside the carboy can force it up and out of place. Keep a close eye on the airlock; when the bubbling subsides, the ferment has started to slow down. After 2 weeks, measure the specific gravity again. When it hits 1.000 to 1.100, the mead is ready for bottling (this final measurement before bottling is the finished gravity, or FG).

6. Secondary fermentation: Prime the bottles with 1 tablespoon honey or about 1 teaspoon priming sugar per 1-quart/1-liter bottle. Pour or siphon the mead into the bottles and seal. Ferment at room temperature for 3 to 5 days, occasionally opening a bottle to check for carbonation. Be careful, as the bottles can explode if there's too much residual sugar in the mead and the bottles are left out for too long (see page 342 for more information on carbonating beverages).

7. Once carbonated, transfer the bottles to the refrigerator or cellar and age the mead for a minimum of 6 months before drinking (1 year is even better). You can drink the mead sooner, but it will just get better with age, and I wouldn't even think of opening it until after the 3-month mark. It will keep for many years, though just as with wine it will eventually peak and decline in quality after aging for many years (decades in some cases).

Note: Lalvin EC-1118 is an excellent Champagne yeast. I love this strain for making higher-alcohol beverages, as well as dry sparkling meads like this one. Lalvin EC-1118 is tolerant of high sugar and high alcohol (18 percent) levels and a wide range of temperatures, from 50° to 95°F.

Fermentation Temperature & Time

Above 75°F
Ferment 3 weeks or less

71° to 75°F
Ferment 3 to 4 weeks

Ideal: 70°F
Ferment 4 weeks

65° to 69°F
Ferment 4 to 5 weeks

Below 65°F
Ferment 5 weeks or more

ELDERBERRY MELOMEL

1,000 grams fresh elderberries, or 500 grams dried

3,200 milliliters filtered water

50 milliliters warm filtered water (75° to 80°F)

1 packet (5 grams) Lalvin 71B-1122 Narbonne yeast (see Note)

1,000 grams light-colored spring honey or other variety (see page 321)

2 grams BSG CraftBrewing Superfood or a comparable yeast nutrient (optional)

EQUIPMENT

Hydrometer

2-gallon or 8-liter (or larger) crock

1-gallon carboy with rubber bung (size 6.5) and airlock

Siphon

Fine-mesh sieve

4 (1-quart or 1-liter) flip-top glass bottles or bottles of your choice, for storage

A melomel is simply a mead which has been fermented with the addition of fruit and/or fruit juice. In all the other mead recipes, the primary fermentation takes place in air-locked carboys; this mead is an example of open-top fermentation. As they do in winemaking, we ferment the must with the fruits for the first 3 to 4 days. The fruit adds flavor, tannins, nutrients for the yeast, and natural sugars, all of which enhance the quality of the finished mead. The addition of fruit also enables you to ferment the mead without using a yeast nutrient (though a nutrient will still enhance and expedite the fermentation and can be added).

Other fresh fruits such as plums, grapes, cherries, or any berry can be used in place of the elderberries in this recipe; just use the same quantity of prepped fresh fruit as you would if using fresh elderberries.

I prefer this mead still, so I ferment until the sugars have all been digested and the mead tastes dry, and then bottle without priming. If you prefer a sparkling mead, prime the bottles and ferment as directed in the recipe for Dry Sparkling Mead on page 328. The longer you age this mead, the better it will get, but if you're quite thirsty, you can drink some of it "green," of course. The last batch of this I made was comparable to any red table wine, with fruity esters and aromas filling the glass. —Shane

1. Wash and sanitize all your fermentation equipment and set aside to air-dry.

2. In a large stockpot, combine the elderberries and the 3,200 milliliters water and bring to a boil. Lower the heat and boil gently for about 30 minutes, until the fruit releases its juices and the must is a dark reddish purple. If using dried berries boil gently for an additional 15 to 30 minutes.

3. Remove the must from the heat, add the honey, and stir to dissolve. Cover loosely with a kitchen towel and allow the must to cool until it reaches a temperature below 80°F. Pour the cooled must into the crock.

4. Meanwhile, to hydrate the yeast, put the 50 milliliters warm water in a measuring cup and pour in the powdered yeast. Let the yeast and warm water stand for 10 to 15 minutes, then stir to combine. (If using a different style of yeast, such as liquid yeast, follow the instructions on the package.) Add the hydrated yeast to the must and stir to combine. Add the yeast nutrient (if using) and stir to combine. Using a wooden spoon, stir vigorously

for 5 minutes (this oxygenates the must, which will facilitate the expedient growth of the yeast). Alternatively, transfer some of the must to a blender and blend for a few minutes to incorporate oxygen, then return the blended must to the pot.

5. Measure the OG of the unfermented must using a hydrometer. Make a note of this number. Cover the crock with a piece of cheesecloth to keep bugs out and secure it with a large rubber band or clean kitchen twine. Ferment the must for 3 to 4 days in a warm place away from direct sunlight. It should be vigorously bubbling by the third or fourth day.

6. Using a siphon, rack the must off the fruit and into the carboy, leaving the neck of the carboy empty, or leaving 3 to 4 inches of headspace. Take the remaining fruit and press it through a fine-mesh sieve to extract as much liquid as you can, and discard the fruit. Ferment the mead in a warm place away from direct sunlight

(4 weeks at 70°F is ideal—see the chart on page 329). Check the bung during the first couple of days, as the pressure building inside the carboy can force it up and out of place. Keep a close eye on the airlock; when the bubbling subsides, the ferment has started to slow down. After 2 weeks, measure the specific gravity again. When it hits 1.000 to 1.100, the mead is ready for bottling (this final measurement before bottling is the finished gravity, or FG).

7. Siphon the mead into bottles, seal, and age the mead in the refrigerator for a minimum of 6 months before drinking (1 year is even better). You can drink the mead sooner, but it will just get better with age, and I wouldn't even think of opening it until after the 3-month mark. It will keep for many years, though just as with wine it will eventually peak and decline in quality after aging for many years (decades in some cases).

Note: Lalvin 71B-1122 is an excellent yeast strain for melomels such as this one. This strain, which was isolated in Narbonne, France, will enhance the flavor of the fruit and also has the ability to metabolize malic acid (a process known as malolactic fermentation), reducing the overall acidity and producing a well-balanced finished beverage. It has a relatively high alcohol tolerance (14 percent) and an ideal temperature range of 60° to 85°F.

APPLE CYSER

50 milliliters warm filtered water (75° to 80°F)

1 packet (5 grams) Lalvin EC-1118 Champagne yeast (see Note, page 329) or Wyeast dry mead yeast (4632)

3,200 milliliters unsweetened apple juice

1,000 grams floral spring honey or other variety (see page 321)

2 grams BSG CraftBrewing Superfood or a comparable yeast nutrient

Honey or sugar (see pages 321, 323), for priming the bottles

EQUIPMENT

Hydrometer

1-gallon carboy with rubber bung (size 6.5) and airlock

Funnel or siphon

4 (1-quart or 1-liter) flip-top glass bottles or bottles of your choice, for storage

Mead that is made with the addition of apple juice is commonly called cyser, and could also be classified as a melomel since it is a mead enhanced with fruit. I've been making hard apple cider for many years now, and it's truly one of my favorite processes. Buying apple juice is fine, but if you really want to take it to the next level, rent an apple press and go glean some apples. People with fruit trees are often quite open to letting you pick their fruit, as long as you ask permission and offer to return the bounty in the form of a couple of bottles of your homemade hooch. In the fall, when apples are bountiful, take note of who in your neighborhood has fruit trees and watch as the apples fall and rot on the ground. We had a number of very prolific apple trees on our property, but I was always able to find other people willing to share their abundance of fruit, which contributes different notes to the finished beverage, as using a variety of apples will produce the best cider.

For this fruity mead, you can use any number of yeast strains. I prefer the Champagne yeast specified in the ingredient list, but you can also use Lalvin ICV-D47 or Wyeast's dry mead yeast (4632). This recipe is intended to produce a dry sparkling mead. If you want a sweeter mead, simply ferment for less time, bottle the mead without priming the bottles, and immediately move the bottles to cellar temperature (50° to 60°F) or into the refrigerator. You can also try using Wyeast sweet mead yeast (4184) instead of the Lalvin EC-1118. —Shane

1. Wash and sanitize all your fermentation equipment and set aside to air-dry.

2. To hydrate the yeast, put the warm water in a measuring cup and pour in the powdered yeast. Let the yeast and warm water stand for 10 to 15 minutes, then stir to combine. (If using a different style of yeast, such as liquid yeast, follow the instructions on the package.)

3. Combine the apple juice and honey in a large stockpot. Add the hydrated yeast and stir to combine. Add the yeast nutrient to the must and stir to combine. Using a wooden spoon, stir vigorously for 5 minutes (this oxygenates the must, which will facilitate the expedient growth of the yeast). Alternatively, transfer some of the

CONTINUED >

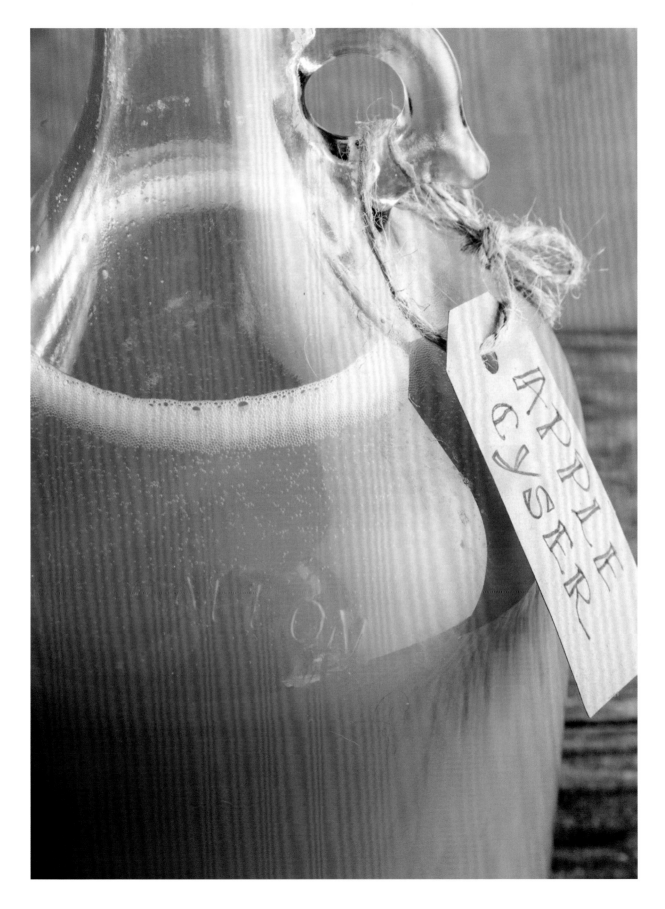

(this final measurement before bottling is the finished gravity, or FG).

7. Secondary fermentation: Prime the bottles with 1 tablespoon honey or about 1 teaspoon priming sugar per 1-quart/1-liter bottle. Siphon the mead into the bottles and seal. Ferment at room temperature for 3 to 5 days, occasionally opening a bottle to check for carbonation. Be careful, as the bottles can explode if there's too much residual sugar in the mead and the bottles are left out for too long (see page 342 for more information on carbonating beverages).

8. Once carbonated, transfer the bottles to the refrigerator or cellar and age the mead for a minimum of 6 months before drinking (1 year is even better). You can drink the mead sooner, but it will just get better with age, and I wouldn't even think of opening it until after the 3-month mark. It will keep for many years, though just as with wine it will eventually peak and decline in quality after aging for many years (decades in some cases).

Fermentation Temperature & Time

Above 68°F
Ferment 3 weeks or less

65° to 68°F
Ferment 3 to 4 weeks

Ideal: 64°F
Ferment 4 weeks

59° to 63°F
Ferment 4 to 5 weeks

Below 59°F
Ferment 5 weeks or more

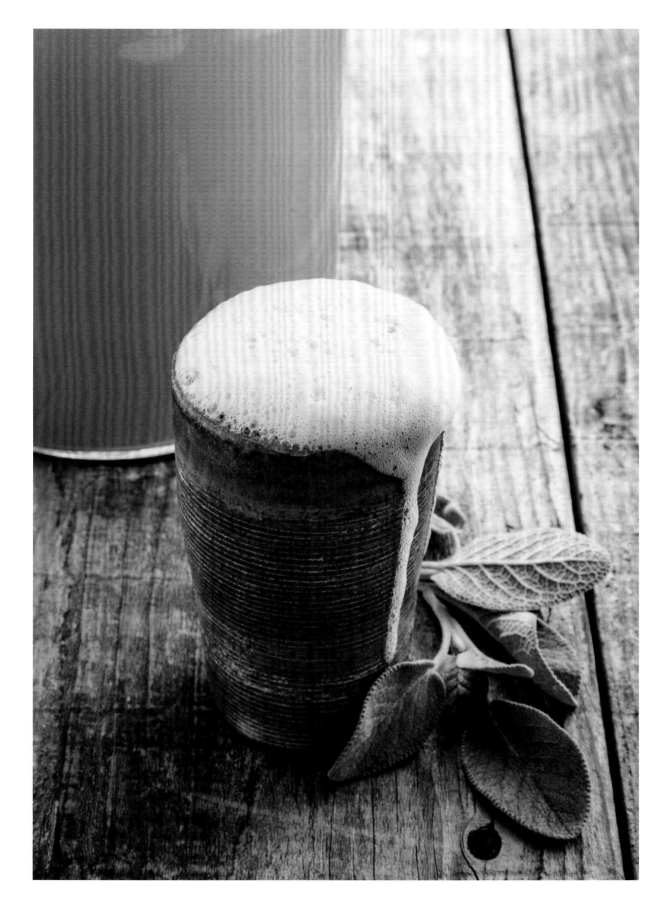

ELDERFLOWER METHEGLIN

400 grams fresh elderflowers (about 1 quart, loosely packed into a jar), or 200 grams dried

1 kilogram floral spring honey

100 milliliters fresh lemon juice (from 2 to 3 lemons)

3,200 milliliters purified or spring water

50 milliliters warm purified or spring water (75° to 80°F)

1 packet (5 grams) Lalvin EC-1118 Champagne yeast (see Note, page 329)

2 grams BSG CraftBrewing Superfood or a comparable yeast nutrient

Honey or elderflower syrup (see page 347), for priming the bottles

EQUIPMENT

Hydrometer

Fine-mesh sieve

1-gallon carboy with rubber bung (size 6.5) and airlock

Funnel or siphon

4 (1-quart or 1-liter) flip-top glass bottles or bottles of your choice, for storage

In the late spring and early summer, forests and fields are filled with the sweet aroma of elderflower, conjuring up images of warmer days to come. One of my favorite ingredients to forage, elderflowers have an unmistakable scent and flavor, reminiscent of a bygone era. In fact, at the time of the American Revolution, elderflower ale was quite a popular beverage, both in the US and in Europe. Although it has fallen out of fashion in most places, in Northern Europe they still drink elderflower-flavored sodas and drinks.

Although it has almost entirely disappeared from American food culture, the elder tree and flowers are out there, probably somewhere near you, waiting to be plucked. Get out into the woods and seek this beautiful plant, for medicinal uses and for food and drink. The berries are also delicious, and while they were once commonly used in pies, jams, and wines, they have fallen into obscurity. Let's bring this beautiful plant back into the mainstream consciousness. As with all foraging, make sure to only take what you need when it is available, and remember that other animals and birds rely on the berries as a food source. If you can't find them or don't want to go to the trouble, you can purchase dried elderflowers online (see Resources, page 348). —Shane

1. Wash and sanitize all your fermentation equipment and set aside to air-dry.

2. Bring the 3,200 milliliters water to a boil in a large stockpot. Remove from the heat. Add the elderflowers and honey and stir to combine. Cover the pot and let steep for 10 to 12 hours. (I like to let the must steep overnight and finish the process the next morning.)

3. To hydrate the yeast, put the 50 milliliters warm water in a measuring cup and pour in the powdered yeast. Let the yeast and warm water stand for 10 to 15 minutes, then stir to combine.

(If using a different style of yeast, such as liquid yeast, follow the instructions on the package.)

4. Strain the must through a fine-mesh sieve set over another stockpot or a large bowl, pressing down on the solids with a wooden spoon to extract all the liquid; discard the solids. Add the hydrated yeast to the must and stir to combine. Add the yeast nutrient to the must and stir to combine. Using a wooden spoon, stir vigorously for 5 minutes (this oxygenates the must, which will facilitate the expedient growth of the yeast). Alternatively, transfer some of the must to a blender and blend for a few minutes to incorporate oxygen, then return the blended must to the pot.

5. Measure the OG of the unfermented must using a hydrometer. Make a note of this number. Transfer the must to the carboy using either the funnel or siphon, leaving the neck of the carboy empty, or leaving 3 to 4 inches of headspace.

6. Ferment the elderflower in a warm place away from direct sunlight (4 weeks at 70°F is ideal—see the chart on page 329). Keep a close eye on the airlock; when the bubbling subsides, the ferment has started to slow down. After 2 weeks, measure the specific gravity—when it hits 1.000 to 1.100, the ale is ready for bottling.

7. Secondary fermentation: Prime the bottles with 1 teaspoon honey or, for additional elderflower flavor, 1 teaspoon elderflower syrup per 1-quart/1-liter bottle. Siphon your brew into the bottles and seal. Ferment at room temperature for 4 to 5 days, occasionally opening a bottle to check for carbonation. Be careful, as the bottles can explode if there's too much residual sugar and the bottles are left out for too long (see page 342 for more information on carbonating beverages).

8. Once carbonated, transfer the bottles to the refrigerator and enjoy. The elderflower will keep for up to 6 months.

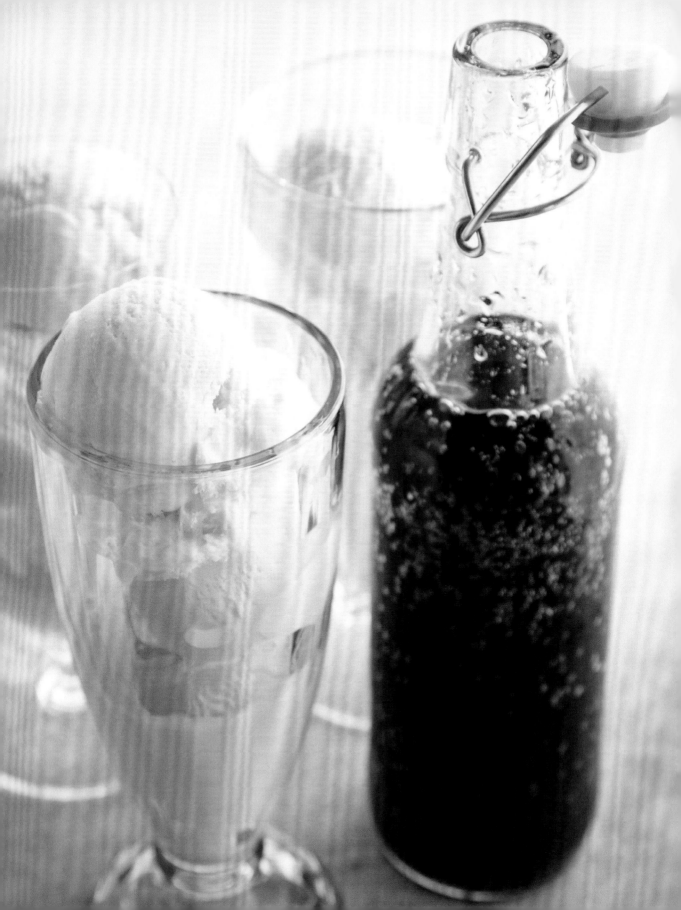

CHAPTER TWELVE

Carbonating and Flavoring Fermented Beverages

This section is intended to shed light on some of the key elements when it comes to carbonating and flavoring your fermented beverages, post-fermentation. You can use all the following techniques to carbonate and flavor your kombucha, water kefir, sour tonics, and alcohol ferments. Adding a sugar source to the bottle prior to adding the ferment is called bottle priming, and the resulting fermentation in the bottle is referred to as a secondary fermentation. Every type of fermented beverage will react slightly different to bottle priming. Some beverages, like water kefir, are very active and can carbonate very fast, especially in warm conditions, whereas others are less active and can take many days to achieve carbonation. This aspect of fermenting beverages could not be easier, as long as you follow a few basic procedures.

There are essentially two methods to carbonate your fermented beverages: you can bottle the fermented liquid while it still has some undigested residual sugar and let it sit at room temperature for a few days so the microbes can digest the remaining sugar and produce CO_2 (which carbonates the beverage); or you can ferment the beverage until dryness, meaning until all the sugar has been digested, then add a priming sugar in whatever form you wish to the bottles before adding the ferment; the microbes will then eat the sugar and produce CO_2. The first method is preferable with beverages like apple cider or sparkling wines, where you're not necessarily trying to get additional flavor into the mix. The second method is better used with ferments such as kombucha and water kefir, or any other fermented beverage to which you want to add more flavor.

Flavoring and carbonation often go hand in hand, because flavoring usually comes in the form of fruit juice, dried fruit, fruit syrups, or herb-infused sugar syrups, all of which give the living microbes in the ferment more sugar to digest, which results in the production of CO_2. You can carbonate your beverages without adding flavoring by bottling the fermented liquid when it still has a little residual sugar or by using a flavorless priming sugar.

There are numerous ways to add flavoring to your fermented beverages. We prefer to add flavoring and carbonation by making concentrated fruit syrups and herb-infused sugar syrups and then adding them to each bottle for a secondary fermentation. The syrups are nice because you don't have to add much to achieve flavor and carbonation simultaneously.

Following you will find our basic syrup recipes and variations, one for making fruit juice syrups and the other for herb-infused syrups. When using these to flavor and carbonate your beverages, the amount you add to each bottle depends on the amount of residual sugar left in the beverage at time of bottling. Tasting is the best way to get a feel for how much syrup to add. Start by adding about a tablespoon of syrup per liter of fermented liquid, taste, and add more if you want a sweeter finished beverage. Let the bottles sit out at room temperature for about three to five days (one to two for water kefir) depending on temperature and amount of sugar used. Once you have done this a few times, you will get a feel for how much sugar to add and how long to ferment for the secondary fermentation. Once carbonated move the bottles to refrigeration where they will continue to ferment, develop flavor, and carbonate at a much slower rate. You can move the primed bottles to refrigeration whenever you feel that they have reached a level of carbonation and flavor that you are satisfied with. Those of you who prefer a sweeter beverage should move the bottles to refrigeration fairly quickly to retain some of the sweetness.

Here are some bottling additions (per 1-liter bottle) that you can use as a rough guide:

- 20 grams dried fruit
- 50 to 100 milliliters fruit juice
- 1 tablespoon fruit or herb-infused syrup
- 1 teaspoon corn sugar or other sugar

Whatever method you choose, be aware of the hazards of overcarbonating your beverages. "Bottle bombs," bottles that explode due to the buildup of CO_2, are a very real danger. I (Shane) have never had a bottle explode in my kitchen, but I've heard some horror stories. You will need to select a bottle that is designed to hold a certain level of carbonation (pressure), such as Champagne bottles, beer bottles, flip-top Grolsch-style bottles, or empty repurposed bottles from store-bought kombucha. There are a few methods you can implement so that you never experience a bottle bomb in your home. One preferred method is to always use one plastic bottle when you bottle a batch of fermented beverages. You can squeeze a plastic bottle to gauge how much pressure is inside and move the bottles to refrigeration when enough CO_2 has been produced but before the plastic bottle is bulging from the pressure. Another method is to add a raisin to each bottle. Initially the raisin will sink to the bottom, but when the beverage is carbonated, it will float to the top.

Again, be very careful not to overcarbonate your fermented beverages, but that being said (and repeated), don't be afraid of flavoring and carbonating your fermented beverages—it's a fun and rewarding aspect of fermentation.

BOILED CIDER SYRUP

MAKES ABOUT 1 PINT

1 gallon apple juice

I started making boiled cider when I was homesteading and had an abundance of apples that we pressed into juice every year. I made hard cider with most of it, but always reserved at least a gallon to make this delicious syrup. This process can be used with any fruit juice to make syrup. The evaporation of the water from the juice really concentrates the flavors and the resulting syrup will make your fermented beverages oh so tasty. This syrup is fantastic for flavoring kombucha, water kefir, and other fermented beverages, and is also delicious on toast with goat cheese, or as an accompaniment to a cheese platter. —Shane

1. Bring the apple juice to a boil in a large stockpot over high heat.

2. Turn the heat to medium-low and simmer the juice until it has reduced to about one-eighth of its original volume (see Note), 1 to 2 hours. (Be careful not to reduce the syrup too far—if you cook the juice to the point that it becomes jamlike, it will still be delicious, but is not ideal for flavoring beverages.) Remove from the heat and set aside to cool until still slightly warm.

3. Transfer the syrup to a jar or bottle, seal, and store in the refrigerator. It will keep for a very long time.

Note: To gauge how much the liquid has reduced, you can periodically pour it into a large measuring vessel (1 gallon of juice reduced to one-eighth its volume is 2 cups or 1 pint). Or use a wooden popsicle stick: Insert the stick in the liquid and mark the starting level on the stick. Place a mark halfway between the starting level and the bottom of the stick, then another mark halfway down from there, and a final mark halfway down from there. Simmer the juice until it has reduced to the lowest mark on the stick.

Variations

You can substitute any other juice for the apple juice to make a wide variety of fruit syrups. Here are some flavor combinations we really like (you can combine the juices in any proportions you like, for a total of 1 gallon):

Blueberry Açai

Ginger Pear

Pineapple Coconut

Cherry Pomegranate

Watermelon Lime

Resources

BREWING SUPPLIES

Adventures in Home Brewing
23847 Van Born Rd.
Taylor, MI 48180
(313) 277-2739
www.homebrewing.org
A great selection of supplies for making beer, wine, and sodas

CROCKS

Harvest Essentials
14525 SW Millikan Way
Beaverton, OR 97005
(503) 828-9820

www.harvestessentials.com/miracle-harsch-gairtopf-fermenting-crock-pots-gartopf.html
German crocks

CULTURES

Amazon
www.amazon.com/Tablespoons-Florida-Sun-Kefir-Organic/dp/B00MK3W3B4
Source for Florida Sun Kefir organic live water kefir grains

Cultures for Health
200 Innovation Ave., Ste. 150
Morrisville, NC 27560
www.culturesforhealth.com

Etsy
www.etsy.com/market/fermentation

Gem Cultures
P.O. Box 39426
Lakewood, WA 98496
(253) 588-2922
www.gemcultures.com

New England Cheese Making Supply Co.
54 Whately Rd.
South Deerfield, MA 01373
(413) 397-2012
www.cheesemaking.com

Weston Price Local Food Chapters
www.westonaprice.org/category/get-involved/local-chapters
Find sources for cultures in your community by joining a local chapter

FERMENTATION EQUIPMENT

Masontops
(800) 353-7258
www.masontops.com
Pickle Pipe fermentation lids

Mountain Feed & Farm Supply
9550 Highway 9
Ben Lomond, CA 95005
(831) 336-8876
www.mountainfeed.com

HIGH-QUALITY HERBS AND SPICES

Monterey Bay Spice Company
241 Walker St.
Watsonville, CA 95076
(800) 500-6148
www.herbco.com

Mountain Rose Herbs
P.O. Box 50220
Eugene, OR 97405
(800) 879-3337
www.mountainroseherbs.com

SaltWorks
16240 Wood-Red Rd. NE
Woodinville, WA 98072
(800) 353-7258
www.seasalt.com

Ohio Stoneware
34 N 3rd St.
Zanesville, OH 43701
(740) 450-4415
www.ohiostoneware.com
American crocks

Stone Creek Trading
Frankfurt, IL
(331) 205-9541
www.stonecreektrading.com/products/fermenting-crock-5-liter
Polish crocks

WEIGHTS

Nourished Essentials
www.nourishedessentials.com/products/the-easy-weight-fermentation-weights-with-grooved-handles
The Easy Weight glass weights

ViscoDisc
www.viscodisc.com
Canning Buddies plastic canning inserts

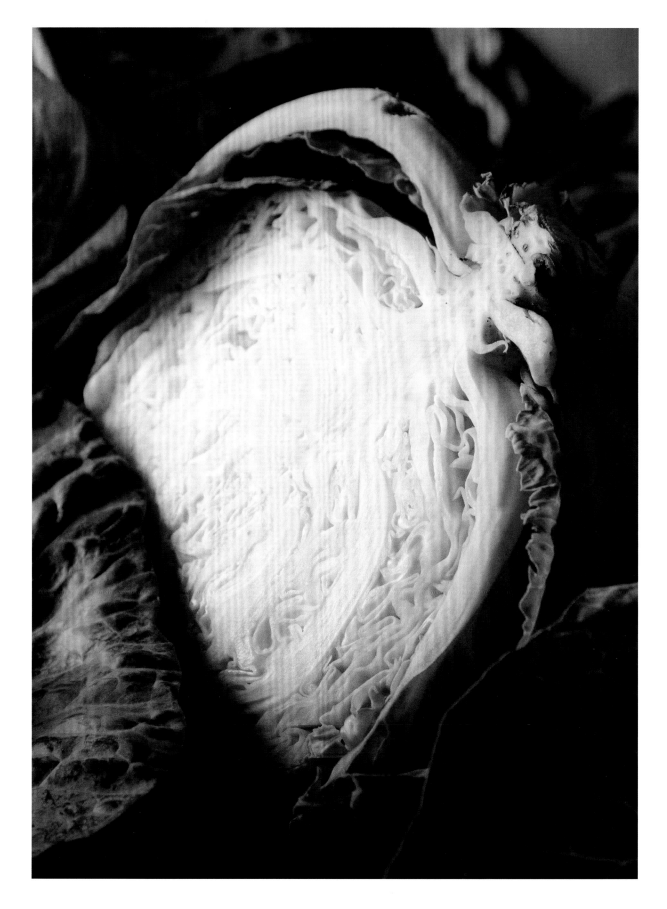

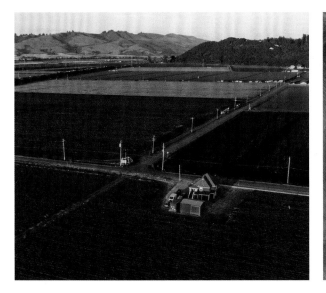

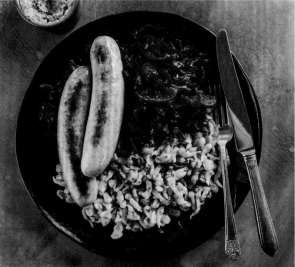

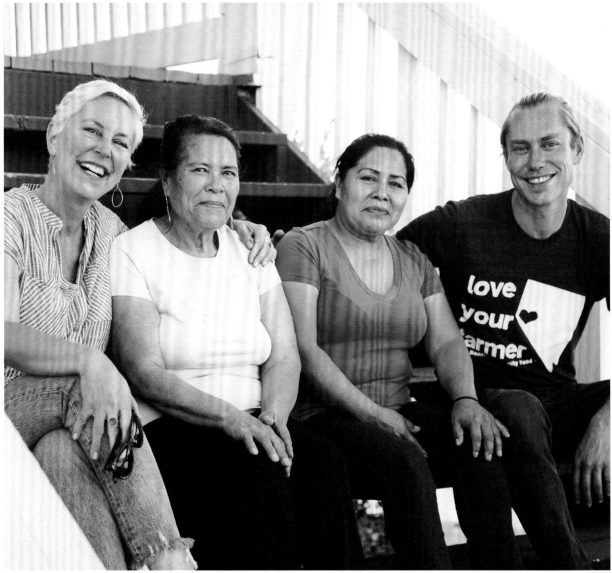

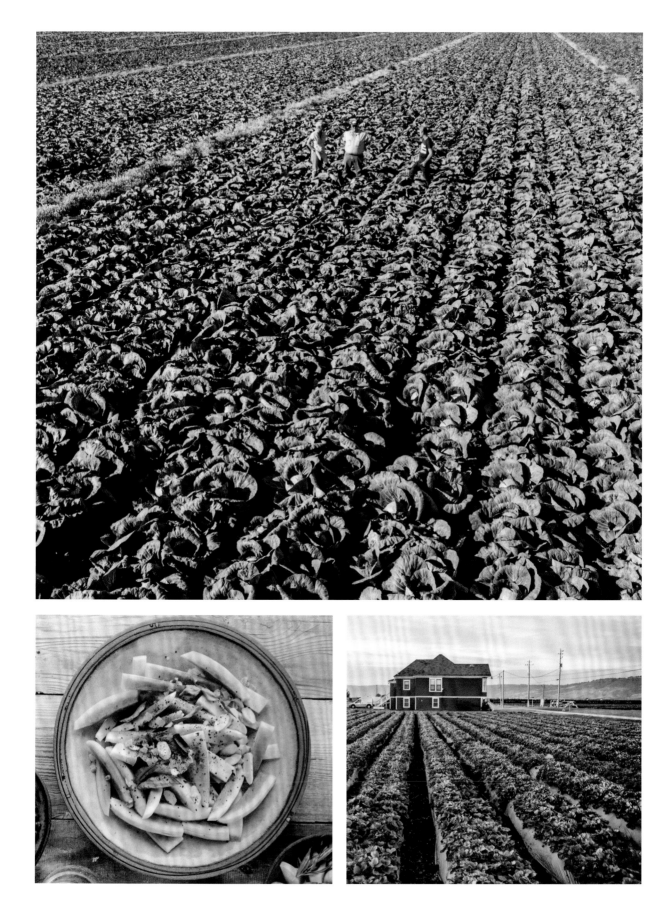

Acknowledgments

The seed for this book was planted more than eight years ago. We desperately wanted to get this information into people's hands so they could feel the same joy we were experiencing with making and eating live culture foods and drinks. But we never quite found the time to birth a book because running the business always took precedence. When we started putting our ideas into a proposal, we quickly realized that the seed planted long ago had not been dormant. In fact it had slowly been germinating through the care and love of so many people.

It all started with Sandor Katz, who is widely considered the godfather of the modern fermentation movement. His fervor, expert advice, and soulful energy are infused into each and every recipe in this book. Thank you for being our spark, Sandor.

While visions of Farmhouse Culture danced in Kathryn's head, David Lukas was her confidant and sounding board. Thank you for your brilliance, David.

When Kathryn began telling family and friends about her crazy idea for a sauerkraut company, a couple of friends were bold enough to pull out their checkbooks to help fund the early days of the business. Our heartfelt appreciation goes out to our angels, Peter Cornelius and Sandy and Hernan Martinez, for their trust and never-failing support through the years.

One of the first employees at Farmhouse Culture was the indomitable Toby Wingo. His ingenuity and kindred connection with the microbial world are very much a part of the Farmhouse Culture DNA. Many thanks are in order for another beloved employee, Doug Beacom. Because of Doug, every bit of our vegetable waste goes to nearby farms for animal feed or compost. Teresa Scalmanani was much more than Kathryn's executive assistant. She was our mother, sister, good friend, and the glue that kept all of us functioning in harmony. Every organization needs a good soldier and at Farmhouse Culture, that person was Kathryn's brother-in-law Jason Lindsay. Thank for you managing our wily farmers' markets through rain and shine and for not calling in sick once in over a decade. And finally a loving shout out to Anita Hernandez who has been with us since 2009. Regardless of the day, Anita always has a smile and a kind word for everyone she meets. She makes all of our days brighter and lighter. Muchas gracias, amiga.

To Kathryn's mother who instructed her in the art of "bad assery." Had she lived to see the birth of the company and this book, she would have been the proudest mother and grandmother on earth. To Kathryn's sister Julianne Boyajian and father Tim Boyajian for their love and support.

Page 350, bottom photo, left to right: Kathryn Lukas, long time Farmhouse Culture employees Anita Hernandez and Maria Isabel Sarate, and Shane Peterson

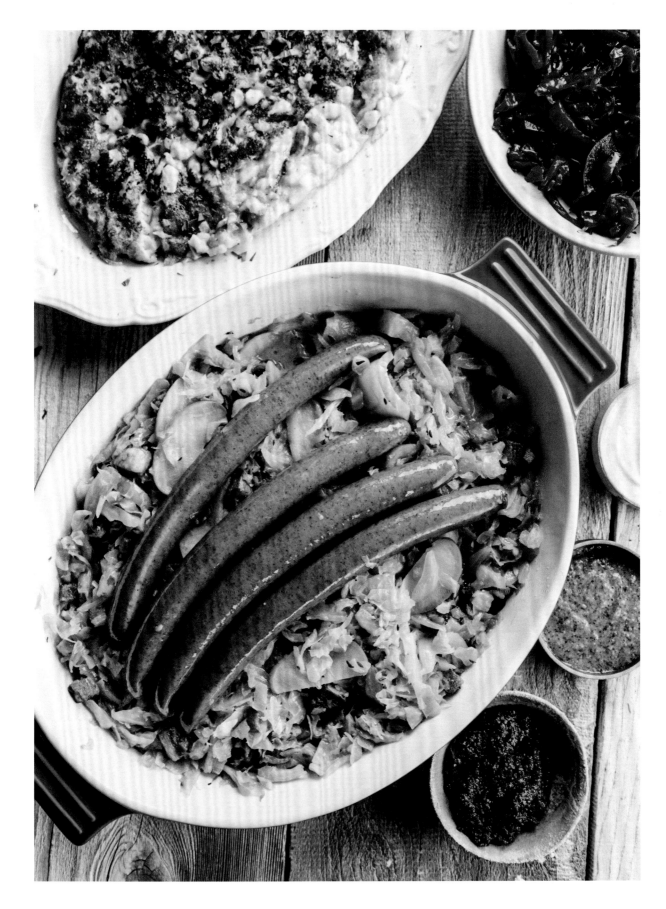

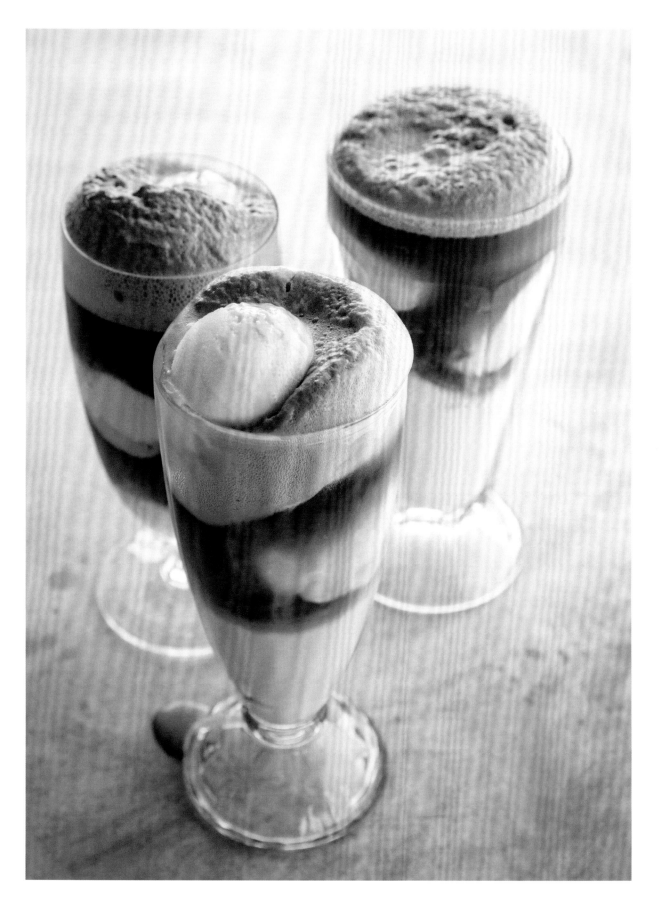

To Jack and Louise Peterson for being the best grandparents in the world to Shane and laying the groundwork for Shane to become a fermenter. Special thanks also go out for the love and encouragement from John Lindsay, Roxanne Hart (RIP), and Leslie Lawton.

To Kirsten Shockey, fermentation expert, bestselling author and Kathryn's Kulture Sister, we thank you for your friendship and the countless hours of bubbly discussion. Much gratitude also goes to Andi and Jorah Roussopoolous, the passionate homestead experts and proprietors at Mountain Feed & Farm Supply, for being our local epicenter of food craft knowledge and for lending preservationist Karla DeLong's expertise when we needed it most.

Thank you Dick Peixoto at Lakeside Organic Gardens for making sure we always had plenty of gorgeous cabbage. A big shout-out to all of you farmers' markets managers who agreed to let us bring our stinky kraut barrels to your markets and also to Harvindar Singh (formerly of Whole Foods Markets), for seeing our potential and putting your card down on the counter at our Slow Food Nation booth in 2008.

As we were developing the proposal for this book, we met the amazingly cheerful and incredibly bright Irene Cho at a food conference in Anaheim where she was marketing the Burma Superstar products and their recent cookbook. Even though Carole Bidnick, the literary agent for their book, was no longer taking new clients, Irene insisted we meet. We did and from the first conversation Carole was kin. But we have no doubt that it was Irene's enthusiastic endorsement that tilted Carole's decision in favor of taking us on. Tragically, Irene passed away unexpectedly in August 2017. We miss you, Irene, and wish you could be here to see your handiwork. Without Carole Bidnick's wise advice, our book proposal may have never landed in front of Jenny Wapner at Ten Speed Press. Thank you Jenny for saying yes. Our heartfelt appreciation also goes out to Dervla Kelly, Kara Plikaitis, Isabelle Gioffredi, Jane Chinn, Allison Renzulli, Kristin Casemore, and managing editor extraordinaire Lisa Regul at Ten Speed Press. Thank you all of your thoughtful guidance and for making this book better than we ever could have on our own. To our epic photographer Eric Wolfinger and his team, *vielen dank* for squeezing us in even though you didn't have time and for making the photos in this book feel as alive as our ferments. And to Eric's incredibly gracious partner Alma for keeping us fed and organized.

We bow in deep gratitude to each and every person who helped us weave this body of work. May it nourish All.

"We don't accomplish anything in this world alone . . . and whatever happens is the result of the whole tapestry of one's life and all the weavings of individual threads from one to another that creates something."

—SANDRA DAY O'CONNOR

Index

kitchen scales, 55
Knight, Rob, 19
kombucha
    about, 300
    fermentation process for, 34–35
    fermenter's notes for, 300–302
    Kombucha Mayo, 305
    master formula for, 306–7
    sour, 304
    Strawberry Kombucha Shrub, 305
    using excess SCOBYs from, 308–9
    vinegar, 304
kosher salt, 59
kraut
    about, 88
    Apple-Fennel Kraut with Red
        Cabbage, 115–16
    Basic Kraut, 92–93
    Chipotle-Lime Kraut with Cacao,
        110–11
    Coyote Kraut, 99–100
    Curried Kraut with Raisins, 97–98
    fermenter's notes for, 88–90
    festivals, 111
    George's Bay Kraut, 112–13
    lacto-fermentation process for,
        24–27
    Miso-Ginger Kraut, 106–7
    Pad Thai Kraut, 102–3
    pink, 83
    softening of, 83–84
    Summer of Love Kraut, 108
    Surf-and-Turf Kraut, 105
    using brine from, 127
kraut tampers, 50
Kuninaka, Akira, 232
Kurlansky, Mark, 56
kvass. *See* sour tonics

L
lactic acid fermentation
    process of, 23–27

starter cultures for, 64–65, 93
Lactobacillus, 25
lag phase, 28, 30
Leach, Jeff, 19
lemons
    Asparagus with Green Garlic and
        Lemon, 228
    Carrot-Lemon Sour, 296
    Julianne's Live Culture
        Lemonade, 103
    Lemon-Ginger Syrup, 347
    Lemon-Tarragon Carrot Sticks,
        229–30
    Preserved Lemons with
        Peppercorns, 278–79
Leuconostoc mesenteroides, 24–25
limes
    Chili-Lime Jicama, 234
    Chipotle-Lime Kraut with Cacao,
        110–11
    Lime-Mint Cucumber Sour, 299
    Spicy Indian Limes, 279
Lindsay, John, 8
Louisiana-Style Hot Sauce, 186–87
Luther, Elaina, 258

M
Mak Baechu–Style Kimchi, 128
mangoes
    Carrot-Coconut Pepper Mash, 197
    Coconut-Mango Water Kefir, 316
Mayo, Kombucha, 305
McGee, Harold, 242, 244
meads
    about, 320–21
    Apple Cyser, 332–34
    Dry Sparkling Mead (Basic
        Hydromel), 328–29
    Elderberry Melomel, 330–31
    Elderflower Metheglin, 338–39
    fermenter's notes for, 321, 323–25
    Sage Metheglin, 335–36

measurements, 55, 76–77, 79
Melomel, Elderberry, 330–31
metheglins
    definition of, 335
    Elderflower Metheglin, 338–39
    Sage Metheglin, 335–36
microbiome, concept of, 18–19
miso
    Miso-Ginger Kraut, 106–7
    Miso-Tamari Pickle Chips, 253
mold, 83
Moroccan Oranges, 279
Morrell, Sally Fallon, 17
mushrooms
    Mushroom Umami Sauce, 232–33
    Surf-and-Turf Kraut, 105
    White Kimchi with Bone Broth and
        Mushrooms, 136–37
mustard
    Beet-Horseradish Mustard, 174
    Horseradish-Mustard Pickles,
        250–51

N
nata, 308
Noma, 48, 232

O
OG (original gravity), 53
onggi pots, 47
Onions, Black Pepper, 175
oranges
    Cranberry-Orange-Walnut Relish,
        268–69
    Date-Orange Water Kefir, 316
    Moroccan Oranges, 279
    Orange-Cardamom Beet Sour, 291
    Orange-Vanilla Syrup, 347

P
Pad Thai Kraut, 102–3
Pasteur, Louis, 16

Peaches, Vanilla-Whey, 270–71
pears
    Ginger-Pear Beet Sour, 295
    Water Kimchi with Asian Pear and
        Pine Nuts, 139–40
Pediococcus, 25
peppers
    Barbados-Style Hot Sauce, 198–99
    Basic Pepper Mash or Hot Sauce,
        184–85
    California-Style Hot Sauce,
        200–202
    Carrot-Coconut Pepper Mash, 197
    Chipotle-Lime Kraut with Cacao,
        110–11
    Coyote Kraut, 99–100
    Eros Pista, 193
    fermenter's notes for, 180–82
    Harissa, 194–95
    Jack's Pickled Peppers, 214–15
    Jamaican-Style Hot Sauce, 192
    Louisiana-Style Hot Sauce, 186–87
    Sambal Bali-Cali, 189–90
    Spicy Chipotle Pickles, 252
    Sriracha, 203
    Sweet Italian Mixed Peppers,
        238–39
    Taco Bar Mix, 210
    Wheezy's Chowchow, 168
Perlmutter, David, 20
Peterson, Jack, 214
pH, measuring, 74–75
pickles
    about, 242–43
    fermenter's notes for, 243–44
    Ginger-Turmeric Pickle Chips, 254
    Half-Sour Garlic Dill Pickles,
        246–47
    Horseradish-Mustard Pickles,
        250–51
    Jack's Pickled Peppers, 214–15
    Miso-Tamari Pickle Chips, 253

Pickled Green Tomatoes, 218–19
    Smoky Tea Pickles, 249
    Spicy Chipotle Pickles, 252
    using brine from, 127
pickling lime, 244
pickling salt, 59
Pine Nuts, Water Kimchi with Asian
        Pear and, 139–40
Pollan, Michael, 18–19, 47
pork, brining, 127
primary fermentation phase, 30–31
probiotic bacteria, 20, 22
Pumpkin Seeds, Kabocha Squash
        Kimchi with, 148–49

R

racking canes, 52
radishes
    Garden Slaw, 165
    Pad Thai Kraut, 102–3
    Ruby Radishes, 213
    Taco Bar Mix, 210
    See also daikon radishes
raisins
    Carrot Kimchi with Raisins, 155
    Curried Kraut with Raisins, 97–98
    Jamaican-Style Hot Sauce, 192
    Swiss-Style Water Kefir, 314–15,
        314–16
Raspberry-Chia Jam, 265
Real Salt, 60
Relish, Cranberry-Orange-Walnut,
        268–69
rice flour, sweet, 125
Robbins, Tom, 222
Rodale, J. I., 17
Root Beer Syrup, 346–47
Root-Chi, 144–45
Ruby Radishes, 213
rutabagas
    Root-Chi, 144–45

S

Saccharomyces cerevisiae, 28, 65
salad dressing, adding brine to, 127
salt
    for brined ferments, 207
    for cucumber pickles, 243–44
    for dry-salted ferments, 158–59
    for kimchi, 124–25
    for kraut, 89
    for preserved citrus, 274–75
    types of, 56–60
SaltWorks, 58
Sambal Bali-Cali, 189–90
sanitization, 71–73
sauces
    adding brine to, 127
    Danish-Style Rémoulade, 162–63
    Mushroom Umami Sauce, 232–33
    See also hot sauces and pepper
        mashes
Scharffenberger, George, 112
SCOBY (symbiotic cultures of bacteria
        and yeast) fermentation,
        34–35, 300
seafood
    Seafood Kimchi, 142–43
    See also shrimp
seaweed
    Surf-and-Turf Kraut, 105
secondary fermentation phase, 31
seedling sprouting mats, 81
shrimp
    George's Bay Kraut, 112–13
    salted, 125
Shrub, Strawberry Kombucha, 305
Sinto Gourmet Kimchi, 111
siphons, 52
Slaw, Garden, 165
Slow Food movement, 6–7
smoked salt, 59
smoothies, adding brine to, 127
son-mat, 26

Published in the United States by Ten Speed Press, an imprint of Random House,
a division of Penguin Random House LLC, New York.
www.tenspeed.com

Ten Speed Press and the Ten Speed Press colophon are
registered trademarks of Penguin Random House LLC.

Library of Congress Cataloging-in-Publication Data
Names: Lukas, Kathryn, 1963- author. | Peterson, Shane, 1983- author.
Title: The farmhouse culture guide to fermenting :
    crafting live cultured foods and drinks with 100 recipes
    from kimchi to kombucha / Kathryn Lukas and Shane Peterson.
Description: California : Ten Speed Press, [2018] | Includes index. |
    Description based on print version record and CIP data
    provided by publisher; resource not viewed.
Identifiers: LCCN 2018038935 (print) | LCCN 2018039354 (ebook) |
    ISBN 9780399582660 (Ebook) | ISBN 9780399582653 (hardcover)
Subjects: LCSH: Fermented foods.
Classification: LCC TP371.44 (ebook) | LCC TP371.44 .L84
    2018 (print) | DDC 664/.024—dc23
    LC record available at https://lccn.loc.gov/2018038935

Hardcover ISBN: 978-0-399-58265-3
eBook ISBN: 978-0-399-58266-0

Printed in China

Design by Isabelle Gioffredi
Food styling by Abby Stolfo
Prop styling by Alma Espinola
All photographs by Eric Wolfinger, except for:
Page 12 from "Food Conservation in North Carolina" by S. R. Winters,
    published in the American Review of Reviews, vol. 56 (November 1917).
Page 18 courtesy of Sandor Katz
Pages 44 and 54 by Amy Spencer

10 9 8 7 6 5 4 3 2 1

First Edition